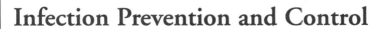

Infection Prevention and Control

Current Research and Practice

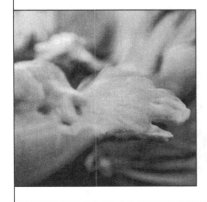

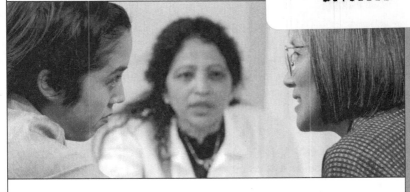

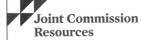

**Joint Commission
Resources**

Joint Commission Resources Mission

The mission of Joint Commission Resources is to continuously improve the safety and quality of care in the United States and in the international community through the provision of education and consultation services and international accreditation.

Joint Commission Resources educational programs and publications support, but are separate from, the accreditation activities of The Joint Commission. Attendees at Joint Commission Resources educational programs and purchasers of Joint Commission Resources publications receive no special consideration or treatment in, or confidential information about, the accreditation process.

The inclusion of an organization name, a product, or a service in a Joint Commission publication should not be construed as an endorsement of such organization, product, or service, nor is failure to include an organization name, a product, or a service to be construed as disapproval.

This publication is designed to provide accurate and authoritative information in regard to the subject matter covered. Every attempt has been made to ensure accuracy at the time of publication; however, please note that laws, regulations, and standards are subject to change. Please also note that some of the examples in this publication are specific to the laws and regulations of the locality of the facility. The information and examples in this publication are provided with the understanding that the publisher is not engaged in providing medical, legal, or other professional advice. If any such assistance is desired, the services of a competent professional person should be sought.

Executive Editor: Paul Reis
Project Manager: Andrew Bernotas
Manager, Publications: Diane Bell
Production Manager: Johanna Harris
Associate Director: Cecily Pew
Executive Director: Catherine Chopp Hinckley
Vice President, Learning: Charles Macfarlane, F.A.C.H.E.

Joint Commission/JCR Reviewers: Peter Angood, Diane Bell, John Cullinan, Catherine Chopp Hinckley, Cecily Pew, Barbara Soule, and Frank Zibrat

Requests for permission to make copies of any part of this work should be mailed to

Permissions Editor
Department of Publications
Joint Commission Resources
One Renaissance Boulevard
Oakbrook Terrace, Illinois 60181
permissions@jcrinc.com

ISBN: 978-1-59940-094-5
Library of Congress Control Number: 2007924655

For more information about Joint Commission Resources, please visit http://www.jcrinc.com.

Contents

SECTION 1: INFECTION PREVENTION AND CONTROL RESEARCH

Dorine Berriel-Cass,
  R.N., M.A., C.I.C
Frank W. Adkins, M.B.A., R.N.

Polly Jones, L.C.S.W., C.P.H.Q.
Mohamad G. Fakih, M.D., M.P.H.

Kimberly J. Rask, M.D., Ph.D.
Linda D. Schuessler, M.S.

Dorothy "Vi" Naylor

Richard P. Shannon, M.D.
Diane Frndak, M.B.A., P.A.-C.
Naida Grunden
Jon C. Lloyd, M.D.
Cheryl Herbert, R.N.

Bhavin Patel, M.D.
Daniel Cummins
Alexander H. Shannon
Paul H. O'Neill
Steven J. Spear, D.B.A.

Marta L. Render, M.D.
Suzanne Brungs, R.N.
Uma Kotagal, M.D.
Mary Nicholson, R.N.
Patricia Burns, R.N.

Deborah Ellis, R.N.
Marla Clifton, R.N.
Rosie Fardo, R.N.
Mark Scott, M.D.
Larry Hirschhorn, Ph.D.

SECTION 2: INFECTION PREVENTION AND CONTROL PRACTICE

ENVIRONMENT

DATA

ASSESSMENT AND PRACTICE

Primum Non Nocere Revisited

Richard P. Shannon, M.D.

Primum non nocere ("First, do no harm") is a tenant of the practice of medicine that provides a succinct and sobering expression of moral principle that encompasses both hope and humility for physicians, particularly those in training. Contrary to popular belief, the phrase does not appear in the Hippocratic Oath, its attribution to Hippocrates is unsubstantiated, and its ori-

About the Author

Richard P. Shannon, M.D. is the Claude R. Joyner Professor of Medicine, Drexel University College of Medicine, and Chairman, Department of Medicine, Allegheny General Hospital, Pittsburgh.

He is also one of the authors of Chapter 3 in this publication, "Using Real-Time Problem Solving to Eliminate Central Line Infections."

gins remain the subject of considerable debate. As the origins of the phrase remain controversial, so too does the meaning . . . to admonish physicians that with the best of intentions may come unwarranted consequences. The modern-day application of this fundamental tenant sits at the heart of the current debate surrounding health care–acquired infections (HAIs) in both the profession and halls of government. It seems HAIs have served to define the modern-day limits of this moral injunction.

Until recently, many in health care believed that the epidemic of HAIs was a regrettable but inevitable consequence of complex care delivered dutifully to eversicker patients. HAIs were collateral damage in the challenging and often-zealous attempt to save human life from the ravages of complex diseases. Yet, both the Institute of Medicine and Centers for Disease Control and Prevention have suggested that we are experiencing a national epidemic of HAIs, raising questions as to what is indeed acceptable. The numbers are staggering and the mortality and costs crippling to a health care system that seems insatiable in its demands for resources.

At the same time, we are witnessing a growing body of evidence that challenges the notion of inevitability and suggests rather that HAIs are a product of unreliable processes and misaligned incentives that reward activity not outcome. These include articles published in *The Joint Commission Journal of Quality and Patient Safety*™ from our program and the work of Peter Pronovost (medical director of the Center for Innovation in Quality Patient Care and an assistant professor in the Department of Anesthesiology/Critical Care Medicine at Johns Hopkins University's School of Medicine) that have demonstrated that certain classes of hospital-acquired infection can be nearly eliminated through the reliable application of existing evidence and refining the care delivery system to minimize unwarranted variation in care delivery. National efforts, such as the Institute for Healthcare Improvement's 100,000 Lives Campaign (and subsequent 5 Million Lives Campaign) have proven similarly what a commitment to address these unsafe conditions can achieve.

A significant factor in support of the theory of inevitability is the fact that we shroud the problem in epidemiological metrics that obscure the human face, thereby mitigating the harm. As an example, in work from our medical intensive care unit and coronary care unit, we were reporting average infections rates of 5.1 infections per 1,000 line-days. But how many human beings did that represent? Five? Ten? Fifty? When the data were presented in such an obscure fashion, we, and I venture to say most health care professionals, were unaware of the tragic human consequences or our own involvement in the events. As a result, it is then easy to dismiss these common occurrences as "unavoidable or inevitable."

The notion of inevitability also has its genesis in the fact that when infections occur, the root cause is not determined immediately. Three or more months after the fact, when the infection is finally reported, the cause of the infection is not apparent, leading to the conclusion that it must be inevitable. Yet, there is no biological basis or genetic mutation that predisposes to HAIs, although there are recognized conditions that pose a greater risk. At the start, I am willing to concede that burn patients, transplant patients, and other immunocompromised hosts are likely at increased biological risk, but this in no way explains the fact that the overwhelming number of reported infections occur in patients without these risks.

Until recently, the best we could do was benchmark against available "norms" such as the National Nosocomial Infection Surveillance data, generating a list of what has become known in safety circles as "the cream of the crap." We now believe that with respect to harmful conditions in health care, the only acceptable benchmark is the pursuit of the theoretical limit. Simply stated: zero infections. The unambiguous goal of zero—that no one should contract an infection in the hospital that they did not have when they arrived—obviates the need for any complex metrics. The argument that normalization of data is necessary to compare hospitals of different sizes and types simply focuses attention on the wrong set of comparisons. The correct approach is for each hospital to demonstrate consistent progress toward the theoretical limit. To those who argue that their patients are sicker, all the more reason to perfect your processes, as no critically ill patient gets better with a superimposed hospital-acquired infection.

In addressing the problem of HAIs, it is useful to look outside our discipline to highly reliable industries that have perfected product development and delivery. There, we see a focus on system redesign that borrows from the wisdom of workers engaged in their practice to gain knowledge as to how processes can be improved. The field of medicine has moved toward embracing the concept of evidence-based practice. While *the evidence* has become increasingly robust, there has been little attention paid to *the practice*—often a chaotic delivery system with unspecified processes and unclear goals—that is the breeding ground for error. Medicine must abandon its hubris and learn from industrial giants that now live the quality dictum as opposed to paying lip service to it.

Needless to say, when you define HAIs as inevitable, you also create the rationale for paying for them. But little is known as to whether hospitals make or lose money when care is complicated by HAIs. Therefore, understanding the economy of HAIs is essential to changing the culture. The current practice that passes commonplace defects along to the purchaser is unsustainable. A national demonstration project performed in all states is required to expose the economic opportunities embedded in the current payments for HAI as part of complexity.

The greatest and certainly most expensive health care system in the world is teetering on the brink of a financial crisis and is becoming an unbearable drag on the nation's economy. The unreliable systems of care delivery and the unsafe conditions that are created as a result undermine the promise of new technology and threaten our ability to afford it. The value added from the elimination of HAIs is more than sufficient to provide insurance for the growing number of uninsured and working Americans, as well as to give us a down payment on the promising new technologies that offer real hope for eradicating disease. Before us lies the first and most important challenge to realize these goals. Are we, as informed citizens and as an honorable profession, willing to commit? Herein lies an equally compelling and sobering Latin aphorism—*cura te ipsum* ("physican, heal thyself"). ■

Foreword

Barbara M. Soule,
R.N., M.P.A., C.I.C.

In 1847 Dr. Ignaz Semmelweis noticed that the women who delivered babies in the hospital ward attended by medical students had high infection rates and deaths after childbirth. As the head of the Maternity Department at the Vienna Lying-In Hospital, Semmelweis was disturbed by the infections and the mortality associated with the childbearing process. In the face of resistance from those who believed that both the puerperal sepsis and related mortality were an inevitable consequence of childbirth, he began to seek the cause for this unacceptable situation. Based on a combination of inductive reasoning, process analysis, scientific assumptions, and keen observation, Semmelweis determined that the infection was carried by the hands of the medical students. He instituted a strict, standardized protocol of hand disinfection for all medical students after they worked on cadavers and before they examined the patients. The mortality rate dropped from 13% to 2% within a year.

About the Author

Barbara M. Soule, R.N., M.P.A., C.I.C., is Practice Leader, Infection Prevention and Control for Joint Commission Resources and Joint Commission International.

During the Crimean War, beginning in 1854, Florence Nightingale spent considerable effort improving the hygiene and cleanliness of the physical environment in the war camp barracks that housed the wounded soldiers. There she found deplorable, filthy environmental conditions that Nightingale believed contributed to illness, and she determined that many injured soldiers were dying from infections rather than their wounds. Nightingale successfully improved sanitation to reduce illness and death in those severe conditions. After returning to England, she used her knowledge and statistics to lobby for better public health measures in health care.

Both of these infection prevention pioneers were successful in their endeavors, due mainly to their strong belief that the infections they observed were not inevitable. Semmelweis and Nightingale were resolute and committed to making a difference and were willing to accept the mantle of leadership required to accomplish the needed changes.

One hundred fifty years later, we continue to face the reality of health care–associated infections (HAIs). By some estimates, the infections are increasing, with a number of organisms becoming more resistant and virulent. The context in which health care is delivered today—and in which HAIs arise—has similarities to the past, along with new and different challenges. Certainly, health care delivery has grown more complex since the 1800s. The systems to provide basic supplies, medications, and other necessities for care are rarely simple and often involve hundreds of steps. It is an ongoing struggle to sustain adequate numbers of qualified personnel, and to maintain a safe physical environment for patients. Efforts to deliver high-quality, effective bedside care are complicated by multiple layers of staff, frequent hand offs, impeded communication, patients moving to many different care settings, and burgeoning regulations.

Amid this complexity, the notion that infections are inevitable outcomes of health care persists, but is gradually changing. The concept of "zero tolerance," is slowly becoming the accepted norm. There is decreasing tolerance among the patients and their families, the public, government, and the media for the seemingly endless reports of hospital infections and deaths and the risk that persons face when they must enter the health care system. What must we do to get this problem under control?

As we struggle to improve seemingly simple processes such as compliance with hand hygiene and environmental safety directives and the more intricate challenges of device-related infections and surgical procedures, we continue to employ approaches similar to those used by Semmelweis and Nightingale. As described in the following pages through the research by Shannon, Render, Berriel-Cass, Rask, Peterson, and their teams, we standardize processes to decrease variability, educate caregivers about their responsibilities, use forcing functions where appropriate, educate staff, and use surveillance metrics to demonstrate progress. The authors have also incorporated newer approaches such as community collaboratives, bundles of evidence-based care practices, rapid action improvement cycles, and groups of care providers who focus on specific improvements. In efforts to reduce infections, a team of professionals may proactively and rapidly respond to a patient with an infection, sometimes as soon as the infection is identified, to analyze the root cause and prevent a future similar occurrence. In addition to these newer interventions, the authors consider the economic costs and potential saving to make the "business case" for up-front outlays for infection prevention efforts, with a sophisticated cost-effective study or a "back-of-the-envelope" analysis. This analysis is often necessary to get the required resources and demonstrate the potential return on investment for preventing infections.

Both Semmelweis and Nightingale believed in using data to characterize the infection risks and to evaluate progress in reducing or eliminating them. The process of monitoring the incidence and prevalence of infections provides the data to guide care decisions and interventions. It lets us know if we are headed in the right direction, toward the "irreducible minimum," or elimination of health care–associated infection as "never" events. Technology increasingly supports efforts to monitor HAIs and demonstrate when improvement activities are successful. Yet much of monitoring continues to be tedious and time consuming. The paper by Gaynes and Platt proposes a case for using valid surrogate measures to save time yet obtain useful data upon which to act.

Lastly, the authors represented in this book unanimously agree that one cannot overestimate the critical role of leadership in contributing to the success of reducing and eliminating HAIs. There appears to be a strong connection between success and leadership's commitment to make the improvement initiatives visible, to allocate the needed resources, to support champions, and to lead the dissemination of successful improvements throughout the organization.

Semmelweis and Nightingale were prominent medical figures of their day. Their brilliant work and subsequent success in reducing infections was shaped by their strong conviction that infections were preventable. They carried out their efforts though sheer determination and unwavering certainty that they could make conditions better for patients. They used the best tools at their disposal and remained committed in the face of resistance and sometimes severe conditions.

Many of the infection challenges of the past remain unresolved, and others have emerged through the years. We have learned new methods from the quality and patient safety movements and from industry and are applying them to reducing infections. Although much has changed in health care delivery, nothing has changed in regard to our responsibility to assure patients of their safety while under our care. Like Semmelweis, Nightingale, and others, we must own the infection problem and persist in finding solutions. Dr. Dennis S. O'Leary, president of The Joint Commission, states "… we all need to come to a clear understanding that there is a problem, that it is a serious problem, and that it is our problem. Then it will become a solvable problem, one commitment, and one step at a time." The authors represented in this book are to be commended for their commitment and excellent work, and we must all join them in finding the solutions for preventing health care–associated infections. ■

Introduction

The numbers don't lie.

Health care–associated infections (HAIs) account for approximately 2 million infections, 90,000 deaths, and $4.5 billion in surplus health care costs each year.[1]

Those numbers and the warnings they bring are being heard by the health care community and beyond. A recent University of Pennsylvania survey of more that 6,300 households showed that 85% of respondents believe knowing a hospital has low infection rates is a very important factor in any hospital-related decision they might make.[2]

However, awareness of infection prevention and control's importance does not mean that everyone is performing their due diligence. A seminal 2001 study published by the Centers for Disease Control and Prevention (CDC) states that despite advances made in infection prevention and control epidemiology and awareness, health care workers' observance of recommended hand hygiene practices—widely considered the foundation of any organization's infection control efforts—is seldom greater than 50%.[3] Some more recent studies indicate higher compliance rates,[4,5] but others show that hand hygiene is not practiced as often as it should be.[6,7]

Infection Prevention and Control: Current Research and Practice is intended to, through its blend of studies and hands-on, common-sense recommendations, serve as a reminder that infection prevention and control (IPC) is a 24-hour-per-day,

365-day-a-year commitment. In the pages that follow, the best of Joint Commission Resources' 2005 and 2006 IPC scholarship documents what has and can still be done to ensure that infections don't happen, or are mitigated when they do.

Richard P. Shannon, M.D., began the book with *"Primum Non Nocere* Revisited," in which he bridged the gulf between "first, do no harm" and "physician, heal thyself."

Barbara M. Soule, R.N., M.P.A, CIC, practice leader, Infection Prevention and Control at Joint Commission Resources, provides her Foreword.

Section 1, "Infection Prevention and Control Research," consists of five studies published in *The Joint Commission Journal on Quality and Patient Safety*™. Each examines different aspects of IPC, from the broad (eliminating infections, patient safety, and surrogate measures) to the specific (central line infections). Central line infections should be of particular interest due to the Institute for Healthcare Improvement's 5 Million Lives Program ("Prevent Central Line Infections" is one of 12 interventions) and because of the possibility of a Joint Commission 2008 National Patient Safety Goal ("Prevent catheter and tubing misconnections") covering this area.

Chapter 1, "Eliminating Nosocomial Infections at Ascension Health" follows St. Louis–based Ascension Health's quest to eliminate HAIs throughout its nationwide network of organizations, starting with St. John Hospital and Medical Center (Detroit, Michigan) and St. Vincent's Hospital (Birmingham, Alabama). The two hospitals used the Institute for Healthcare Improvement model of "bundles" to achieve the goal of reducing HAIs and also implemented multidisciplinary rounds and the use of daily goal sheets in the intensive care unit.

Chapter 2, "A Statewide Voluntary Patient Safety Initiative: The Georgia Experience," explores the work of the Georgia-based Partnership for Health and Accountability (PHA), a voluntary quality improvement and patient safety program consisting of the Georgia Hospital Association and 75 stakeholder organizations focused on comprehensive evaluation and feedback. PHA provides access to quality and safety tools and benchmarking resources for a diverse group of hospitals, including rural and critical access facilities. Case studies of two organizations bear out PHA's efforts to encourage improvement and flexibility in an atmosphere of changing patient-safety priorities.

Chapter 3, "Using Real-Time Problem Solving to Eliminate Central Line Infections," details the efforts of two intensive care units (ICUs) employing the principles of the Toyota Production System to reduce central line–associated bloodstream (CLAB) infections. New processes produced significant CLAB infection decreases within one year (from 10.5 to 1.2 infections/1,000 line-days), and even more drastic decreases in mortalities (from 19 to 1), despite an increase in the use of central lines and number of line-days.

More work with central lines is featured in Chapter 4, "Evidence-Based Practice to Reduce Central Line Infections." In 2003 nine Cincinnati-area health care systems took part in a two-year project to reduce central line infections among patients in ICUs and following surgery. All reduced central line infections by 50% due to the direct role of hospital leadership, development of a local community of practice, the cooperation of physicians, and problem solving.

Chapter 5, "Monitoring Patient Safety in Health Care: Building the Case for Surrogate Measures," discusses a new approach to monitoring the measurement of adverse events, based on experience in measuring hospital-associated infections. The authors argue that developing clinically relevant processes or surrogate measures that clinicians would use to improve patient outcomes is essential.

Chapter 6, "Modifying the Universal Protocol for Effective Delivery of Perioperative Prophylactic Antibiotics," describes one hospital's improvement in the process of antibiotic delivery by leveraging compliance with The Joint Commission's Universal Protocol for Preventing Wrong Site, Wrong Procedure, Wrong Person Surgery™.

Section 2, "Infection Prevention and Control Practice," includes a variety of practice- and example-driven chapters grouped by three subject areas: "Environment," "Data," and "Assessment and Practice."

The "Environment" section is comprised of three chapters: Chapter 7, "Private Rooms and the Environment of Care: Organizations Recognizing Safety and Privacy Benefits of Single-Patient Rooms," an examination of patient safety in an era of increasing requests for private rooms; Chapter 8, "Building Contractor Awareness: One Hospital Uses a Handbook to Help Educate Construction Workers," one organization's attempt to bring its construction personnel under the patient safety "umbrella"; and Chapter 9, "Preparing for a Pandemic: Infection Control Experts Discuss Avian Flu—and Not 'Whether' but 'When,'" a discussion by avian flu experts on the probability of a significant outbreak of that disease and how to take steps to minimize such an occurrence.

The two articles on "Data" display the importance of surveillance of organizational performance to patient safety. Chapter 10, "Surgical Care Infection Prevention Data Are Collected to Reduce Incidence of Surgical Complications," explains some of the surgical care infection prevention data analysis available to organizations and the general public via The Joint Commission's Quality Check® Web site. Chapter 11, "National Data Report: Hospital Infection Reporting Guidelines," outlines the current state of infection reporting for U.S. hospitals and outlines the CDC's recommended measures for HAI disclosure.

"Assessment and Practice," the book's final section, concentrates on practical, hands-on tips for evaluating and improving your organization's infection prevention and control performance. Chapter 12, "Ensuring the Use of Sterilized and Disinfected Equipment: Improving Infection Control While Reducing Turnaround Time and Costs," provides five practical, straightforward tips for safe, time-efficient infection control. Chapter 13, "Assessing and Addressing Infection Control Risks: How Does Your Organization Measure Up?" gives your organization a road map for developing and implementing an effective infection prevention and control plan. Chapter 14, "How Well Does Your Organization's Infection Control Program Work?" uses Joint Commission standards as a basis for organizational self-evaluation. Chapter 15, "Making the Business Case for Infection Control," points out that although patient safety should be at the core of all health care decisions, effective infection control and prevention makes sense as a cost-cutting agent as well.

A detailed index is also included.

Special thanks to Rick Shannon and Barb Soule for their excellent work on this book's front matter. Thanks also to Dr. Shannon and all of the other authors of the six studies that form Section 1 of this book. Special thanks to Pam Brick for her work updating and reorganizing Section 2, and to reviewers Peter Angood, Diane Bell, John Cullinan, Cathy Hinckley, Cecily Pew, Barb Soule, and Frank Zibrat for their input and support. ■

References

1. Weinstein R.A.: Nosocomial infection update. *Emerg Infect Dis* 4:416–420, 1998.

2. McGuckin M., Waterman R., Shubin A.: Consumer attitudes about health care–acquired infections and hand hygiene. *Am J Med Qual.* 21:342–346, Sep.–Oct. 2006.

3. Pittet D.: Improving adherence to hand hygiene practice: A multidisciplinary approach. *Emerg Infect Dis* 7:234–240, Mar.–Apr. 2001.

4. Randle J., Clarke M., Storr J.: Hand hygiene compliance in healthcare workers. *J Hosp Infect* 64:205–209, Nov. 2006.

5. Lam B.C., Lee J., Lau Y.L.: Hand hygiene practices in a neonatal intensive care unit: A multimodal intervention and impact on nosocomial infection. *Pediatrics* 114:e565–e571, Nov. 2004

6. Amazian K., et al.: Multicentre study on hand hygiene facilities and practice in the Mediterranean area: Results from the NosoMed Network. *J Hosp Infect* 62:311–318, Mar. 2006.

7. Patarakul K., et al.: Cross-sectional survey of hand-hygiene compliance and attitudes of health care workers and visitors in the intensive care units at King Chulalongkorn Memorial Hospital. *J Med Assoc Thai* 88 (suppl 4):S287–S293, Sep. 2005.

SECTION 1

Infection Prevention and Control Research

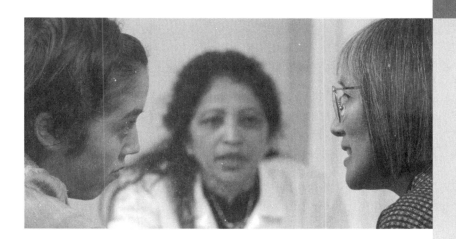

Eliminating Nosocomial Infections at Ascension Health

Dorine Berriel-Cass, R.N.,
M.A., C.I.C.
Frank W. Adkins,
M.B.A., R.N.

Polly Jones, L.C.S.W.,
C.P.H.Q.
Mohamad G. Fakih,
M.D., M.P.H.

As described elsewhere,[1,2] Ascension Health, the largest Catholic and largest nonprofit health care system in the United States, has articulated a call to action that promises to provide "Healthcare That Works, Healthcare That Is Safe, and Healthcare That Leaves No One Behind, for Life," and to the goal of excellent clinical care with no preventable injuries or deaths by July 2008. This article reports on two alpha sites' experience in addressing one of Ascension Health's priorities for action—nosocomial infections.

About the Authors

Dorine Berriel-Cass, R.N., M.A., C.I.C., is Manager, Infection Control, St. John Hospital and Medical Center, Detroit.

Frank W. Adkins, M.B.A., R.N., is Affinity Group Project Manager, St. Vincent's Hospital, Birmingham, Alabama.

Polly Jones, L.C.S.W., is Director, Clinical Excellence, Ascension Health, St. Louis.

Mohamad G. Fakih, M.D., M.P.H., is Medical Director, Infection Control, St. John Hospital and Medical Center.

Please address correspondence to Mohamad G. Fakih, Mohamad.Fakih@stjohn.org.

Nosocomial infections comprise one of the leading causes of preventable injuries and deaths in hospitals, affecting 5% to 10% of hospitalized patients and contributing to increased morbidity, mortality, length of stay, and cost.[3-5] Catheter-related bloodstream infections (CR-BSIs) and ventilator-associated pneumonia (VAP) account for the most significant morbidity, mortality, and cost.[3] Although nosocomial infections historically have been accepted as adverse events related to hospitalization, they are considered preventable; therefore, a lower rate of nosocomial infections is a reflection of a higher quality of care. Compliance with evidence-based guidelines for preventing CR-BSIs and VAPs[6,7] is not universal, and variation of practice is still common.

Risk Factors and Prevention Measures

The risk for CR-BSI starts with the insertion of the catheter. Both phlebitis and septicemia can occur with a peripheral intravenous (IV) catheter, as well as with a central venous catheter, also known as a central line (CL). Although these complications can occur with both peripheral and CLs, the prevalence is higher with CLs.[8] The subclavian site is recommended as the preferred site because it is associated with a lower risk of infection.[6] The femoral site has been discouraged because of a higher incidence of infectious and thrombotic complications.[3,9] Most of the early-onset infections occur because of poor compliance with hand hygiene and/or aseptic technique that call for maximum sterile barriers and chlorhexidine disinfection.[3,10] A process that incorporates hand hygiene, antiseptic techniques, and use of maximum barrier precautions should lead to a reduction in CR-BSIs.

VAP is defined as a pneumonia that develops more than 48 hours after endotracheal intubation, affects 8% to 28% of those on mechanical ventilation, and is associated with high mortality (25%–50%).[11–13] It also is associated with increased morbidity, length of stay (LOS), and cost, which may reach $40,000 per case.[11–13] Risk factors for VAP include nonmodifiable and modifiable factors.[12] Host factors, which are difficult to alter, include older patients, high severity of illness, altered mental status, and chronic pulmonary disease. However, attention to intervention and treatment factors will help reduce the rate of VAP.

Multiple interventions have shown benefit in reducing the risk of VAP, including avoiding tracheal intubation and using noninvasive positive pressure ventilation, shorter duration of mechanical ventilation, subglottic suctioning, avoiding nasal intubation, and avoiding manipulation of ventilatory circuit.[11] Placing intubated patients in the semirecumbent position, avoiding stomach distention or gastric residuals, and maintaining oral hygiene have contributed to a lower VAP rate.[11–13]

Reducing CR-BSI: The SJHMC Experience

St. John Hospital and Medical Center (SJHMC), a 607-bed tertiary-care teaching facility in Detroit, has 60 adult critical care beds across four units: surgical (SICU), medical (MICU), cardiac (CICU), and cardiovascular ICU (CVICU). Intensivists and resident physicians manage patients in the ICUs. In 2003, CL use (CL days/patient days) ranged from 42% to 98%. Although most of these CLs were inserted in one of the four ICUs, some were placed in the operating room (OR), emergency department (ED), or on the general nursing unit. Intensivists and attending and resident physicians insert CLs.

Nurses assist the physicians with line insertion by gathering supplies and preparing IV setups. Nosocomial surveillance for CR-BSI is conducted by infection control practitioners (ICPs) using the National Nosocomial Infections Surveillance System (NNIS) definitions.[14] In 2003, SJHMC's CR-BSI rate averaged 7.0 (range, 4.3–9.0) per 1,000 CL days. An opportunity existed to improve patient safety by decreasing the risk of CR-BSI.

DEVELOPING THE TEAM

The initiative began in February 2004, when Ascension Health accepted SJHMC's proposal to become an alpha site for reducing nosocomial infections. Alpha sites were selected on the basis of local leadership's commitment to the initiative and willingness to allocate human and other resources to complete small tests of change in the designated focus area, evaluate the effect, track improvements, and lead the spread of successful strategies throughout the system. Each alpha site was allowed to choose its priority for action.

The rate of CR-BSIs in the ICUs was higher than NNIS rates, and efforts were initiated to reduce infection. A more structured approach to improve the process was needed. The infection control department met with the senior vice president of quality and the hospital chief executive officer (CEO) to describe the process to improve patient care and reduce costs. Senior leadership's support was key to ensuring availability of resources and enhancing the visibility of the initiative.

DEVELOPING THE CL BUNDLE

The infection control department put together the educational component for physicians and nurses, with its medical director [M.G.F.] providing the education to physicians, and the ICPs providing it to nursing. In addition, ICPs educated rotating resident physicians in the ICU monthly. The educational program addressed the following:

- The significance of the problem with CR-BSI, the associated morbidity and mortality, and its financial impact on hospitals

- Types of CLs, indications for their use, and associated risk (infectious and noninfectious), included alternate-access catheters with lower risk (peripherally inserted central catheters or peripheral intravenous catheters if no central access was required).
- Appropriate site of placement with a focus on avoiding femoral lines, a technique supported by our hospital policy, which discourages the use of femoral lines except for cases with high risk for pneumothorax and risk of noncompressible hematoma. Routine change or exchange over a guide wire of CL was discouraged.
- NNIS definitions of CR-BSI
- Detailed description of the tools for the procedure, including the CL cart, CL kit, CL checklist, and CL bundle components; this included a detailed description of the appropriate procedure for applying chlorhexidine and dressing changes.
- Tools to assess compliance (reviewing the checklist for documentation of compliance with the required bundle components)
- Measurement of outcomes (CR-BSI)
- Addressing potential barriers with implementation
- Promoting the role of the IV team in CL care

A protocol for line insertion was identified through the use of Centers for Disease Control and Prevention Healthcare Infection Control Practices Advisory Committee guidelines[6] and the Institute for Healthcare Improvement (IHI) Central Line Bundle Mode.[15] Best practices were identified as skin preparation with a chlorhexidine product and use of a full sterile drape to cover the patient. In addition, physicians placing CLs were required to practice hand hygiene before insertion and wear a sterile gown, gloves, and cap/mask. A checklist was developed for CL insertions that would be utilized to assess compliance with this protocol. The checklist included the following items:

- Before the procedure: hand hygiene by physician, the use of chlorhexidine, and use of a full drape
- During the procedure: use of hat, mask, and gown, maintenance of a sterile field, and the use of the assistant in the procedure of the same precautions
- After the procedure: application of a sterile dressing

The checklist forced compliance with the components of the procedure by not allowing the operator to proceed without following the best practices. The checklist did not allow "no" as one of the answers. The two options were either "yes" or "yes after correction."

Nursing and physician champions were designated. The nursing champion was defined as a nurse well known in the ICU who was involved in training nurses on his or her unit on using the checklist to document the correct placement of central catheters and was responsible for compliance with the checklist on all lines placed. The unit nurse manager acted as the nurse champion and supported the nurses' stopping of the procedure at any time if the physician was not complying with the established protocol. The physician champion was chosen based on being well known in the ICU, being involved in training residents for catheter placement, directing in-services for resident physicians (medical and surgical) on appropriate line placement and the use of the tool, and serving as a contact person if problems occur between operator (physician) and nursing. The ICU's medical director was asked to be the physician champion and was directly contacted if there were any issues with the procedure.

A CL insertion cart containing necessary supplies was assembled, including the chlorhexidine skin preparation product, which was new to the ICUs. Before starting the intervention, a gap analysis was conducted to identify deficiencies between current practice and the new protocol (*see* Table 1-1). The CL kit was customized to include a large drape and chlorhexidine gluconate for skin antisepsis.

A team consisting of an ICP, medical director of infection control, and the IV nursing manager developed a plan for line tracking, dressing changes, and facilitating removal of the CL.[15] The team met with information technology to develop an electronic database for tracking CLs. The goal was to follow all CLs placed in ICU and promote their discontinuation when they were no longer necessary, even after the patient's transfer from ICU.

IMPLEMENTATION AND MEASUREMENT

The new protocol was started with one nurse, one physician, and one patient. This process was then spread to involve all patients and nurses in the pilot ICU, and eventually all the ICUs were involved. Throughout the initiative, the ICPs rounded in the ICUs daily to collect the checklist and provide feedback if the form was

TABLE 1-1. St. John Hospital and Medical Center's Gap Analysis of Central Line Bundle Components

Central Line Bundle	Yes*	No†
Product for hand hygiene	X	
Chlorhexidine gluconate for skin antisepsis		X
Full sterile drape		X
Physician wears sterile gloves/ gown, cap, and mask		X Gown and cap not always worn
Avoid femoral lines	X Policy addresses issue	
Sterile dressing applied	X	
* Already in place † Needs to be implemented		

Source: Authors.

missing information or not completed correctly. All components of the bundle needed to be present, or the operator was considered noncompliant. The information from the checklist was then entered into the database. The checklist was revised three times to make it user friendly and still capture key information. Multidisciplinary rounds (MDR) were incorporated into the ICU practice before the initiative; however, use of the daily goal sheet was new to the process. The sheet served as a communication tool regarding the plan of care for each ICU patient.

Monthly CR-BSI rates were reported back to the individual ICUs. Unit rates were compared with historical and NNIS rates[14]; feedback was important to maintain momentum.[6] Each report included high-level detail regarding the use of the protocol for line insertion. CR-BSI rates were also included on the hospital scorecard. Several months into the initiative, the CEO sponsored a celebration for the ICU nursing staff to recognize its efforts.

Data on daily CL utilization were collected through our ICU surveillance of all CLs (including Swan-Ganz, short-term triple-lumen catheters, and peripherally inserted CLs). The involved units submitted daily reports to infection control indicating the number of patients with a CL. All patients in ICU with positive blood cultures were evaluated by the ICPs for potential CR-BSIs.

Results

CR-BSI rates were compared pre- and postintervention. The CR-BSI rate gradually decreased in the ICUs. The initial goal was to reduce CR-BSIs in the ICUs by 30%. Before the intervention (July 2003–January 2004), the mean CR-BSI rate was 9.6 per 1,000 catheter days. The mean CR-BSI rate since the start of the intervention (February 2004–January 2006) was 3.0 per 1,000 catheter days—significantly lower than preintervention rates (independent 2-tailed t-test, assuming different variances, $p = .003$). In the first year of the intervention (February 2004–January 2005), CR-BSIs were reduced by 55%, exceeding the goal. Figure 1-1 shows the decrease in the CR-BSI rate in the SICU, our pilot unit. In the first year of implementation in the pilot ICU, 92% (438/474) of the CLs were placed using the bundle.

Detailed analysis of each CR-BSI allowed the team to determine if it was a potentially avoidable infection. When we reviewed CR-BSIs, we determined if the CL bundle was used for line insertion. Eleven (73%) of the 15 cases with CR-BSIs did not have documentation of the use of the CL bundle. The ICPs found that for some of the CR-BSIs, the CL was placed outside the ICU, in an area of the hospital not using the bundle, including the OR, ED, and medical-surgical general units. These data provided the opportunity to spread the learning experience from the ICUs to other areas of the hospital to standardize the safest practice throughout the facility.

Implementation of the CL bundle was associated with a longer period of infection-free catheter days in ICU patients placed on the bundle. For patients with CR-BSI, the average time to acquire infection increased from 5.8 days in 2004 to 13.2 days in 2005. Catheter manipulation or site care may be the contributing factors to these infections.[16] A program is being developed to reinforce ongoing CL care. In addition, we promoted the use of lower-risk devices such as peripherally inserted central catheters for those who need long-term IV access or peripheral IV catheters if appropriate.

We encountered barriers in developing and maintaining an electronic database to track CL. The IV team nurses were asked to input the data and follow up on all

FIGURE 1-1. St. John Hospital and Medical Center SICU CR-BSI Rate, July 2003–January 2006

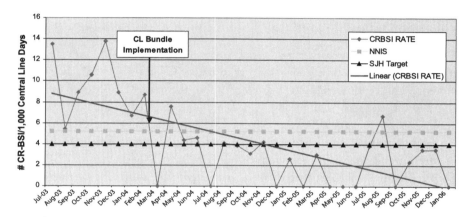

Surgical (SICU) catheter-related bloodstream infection (CR-BSI) rates at St. John Hospital and Medical Center (SJH) are shown in comparison with historical mean (diagonal line) and National Nosocomial Infections Surveillance System (NNIS) rates. CL, central line.
Source: Authors.

patients transferred from ICU with a CL. The IV team manager was supportive, but initial resistance was noted by many IV team nurses. The system was seen as complicated and not user friendly. Although the IV team nurses rounded on all medical-surgical units, they never intervened to discontinue unnecessary CLs on the general wards. With the encountered resistance by the IV team nurses, this effort was later halted.

Reducing VAP: The STV Experience

St. Vincent's Hospital (STV), a 338-bed acute-care hospital in Birmingham, Alabama, that serves a five-county area, has two 14-bed ICUs (medical-surgical ICU and CVICU). The medicalsurgical ICU, which served as the pilot for the initiative to eliminate VAP, is the focus for this article.

STV does not have an intensivist program, and most patients on mechanical ventilation at STV are managed by pulmonary physicians. Respiratory therapy and nursing assist in managing these patients, and the infection control manager performs surveillance for VAP, using the NNIS definitions.[14] For the 13 months before the intervention, the average rate of VAPs in ICU was 8.2 per 1,000 ventilator days—higher than the NNIS pooled mean of 5.4.

DEVELOPING THE TEAM

In February 2004, STV started its project to reduce nosocomial infections, working with Ascension Health and the IHI Critical Care Collaborative.[17] The administration committed its financial support of the project. A team of ICU nurses, representatives from administration, and quality managers was formed. Concepts introduced included use of bundles, MDR, daily goal sheets, small tests of change, and measurement of results. An implementation team, established to develop the process changes and further define goals, included nursing staff, pharmacy, infection control, case management, social workers, dietary, respiratory, chaplain, transporters, quality managers, and a representative from CVICU, who would eventually spread the process changes to that unit. The team was designated the MDR team and served as the catalyst to the changes. Although the long-term goal was to reduce the number of VAPs to zero, the immediate goals established by the MDR team associated with VAP were as follows:

- Reduce the VAP rate by 50%.
- Reduce the number of ventilator days by 50%.
- Reduce the average number of days a patient was mechanically ventilated by 50%.
- Reduce ICU LOS by two days.

Staff education was a necessary component at each step in the process change. The MDR team ensured staff's understanding of all aspects of the changes to come. Impediments to educating all staff included the use of traveling nurses and temporary staff and the normal turnover rate among staff nurses. A train-the-trainer approach was taken to accomplish the necessary staff education. Charge nurses, who were educated first, educated the staff on their various shifts. ICU managers attended the nurse orientation program to explain the MDR, bundles, and other changes occurring in the critical care environment. The same approach was used with all new employees and with continuing education for staff.

Physicians were educated on the changes under way and were encouraged to participate. Although there was a lot of interest among the physicians, there was limited direct participation by them initially.

DEVELOPING THE VENTILATOR BUNDLE

The MDR team designed a daily goal sheet, developed a VAP bundle, defined methodology for data collection and reporting, and determined an implementation date. The MDR team's role was critical to the overall success in implementing the changes.

The daily goal sheet became the MDR team's standardized tool (although one that can be revised as needed) for communication about the ICU patient. It included the elements of the VAP bundle, as well as other supportive evaluations, and provided a good overview of the patient's condition on that day. It was used to document recommended changes that needed to be communicated to the physician and other MDR team members, and finally, what was needed to transfer patients out to the medical-surgical units to improve flow.

The MDR team developed the bundle for ventilator patients on the basis of IHI guidelines.[17] The initial bundle consisted of head of the bed (HOB) at 30 degrees, deep vein thrombosis (DVT) prophylaxis, peptic ulcer disease (PUD) prophylaxis, oral care every two hours, and hand washing[7] (see Table 1-2). Two other suggested bundle elements—sedation vacation and weaning protocol—were not implemented initially. However, protocols were developed later for each, and STV is moving toward implementation.

HOB. HOB at 30 degrees was the first bundle element implemented. An observation survey by the MDR team revealed that the ICU beds were elevated around 10–15 degrees. Measurement by the staff nurse was made easy with incorporation of a bubble protractor that indicated HOB elevation in the ICU beds. In addition, ICU beds supporting mechanically ventilated patients had pressure relief surfaces, therefore minimizing the risk for pressure ulcers.

DVT. Patients with respiratory failure have an increased risk of developing a DVT. Studies show that 22%–80% of ICU patients develop a DVT because of prolonged immobility, sepsis, and vascular injury from indwelling catheters or other invasive devices.[18] All ICU patients were placed on DVT prophylaxis, unless contraindicated.

TABLE 1-2. St. Vincent's Hospital's Ventilator and Oral Care Bundles

Ventilator Bundle	Oral Care Bundle
• Head of bed at 30 degrees	• Oral care every 2 hours
• Deep vein thrombosis prophylaxis	• Use suction toothbrush 0800 and 2000
• Peptic ulcer disease prophylaxis	• Suction secretions from the back of throat before performing
• Sedation vacation	• Use suction swabs with peroximint except at 0800 and 2000 when suction toothbrush is used
• Daily weaning trial	• After each 2-hour oral suctioning, apply moisturizer to all mucous membranes, gums, and patient's lips
• Oral care bundle	• Document in nursing notes

Source: Authors.

PUD. Patients with respiratory failure who are mechanically ventilated have an increased risk for developing stress ulcers and associated gastrointestinal bleeding. Factors that affect this include decreased gastric pH, increased gastric mucosal permeability, and ischemia.[19] Patients with a nasogastric tube show a significantly higher risk of developing gastrointestinal bleeding independent of body position.[20] Patients requiring ventilator support were placed on PUD prophylaxis on intubation.

IMPLEMENTATION AND MEASUREMENT

The ICU staff nurse measured DVT and PUD prophylaxis compliance and reported findings in the daily MDR meeting. If no order was obtained for the appropriate prophylaxis, the staff nurse followed up with the physician to determine why prophylaxis was omitted.

Kits containing the material for every-two-hour oral care were placed in the patient room each morning and inventoried the next day by the staff nurse to determine use. Compliance was reported in the daily MDR meeting.

Hand washing was the most difficult part of the bundle to measure. Different methods were used in an attempt to obtain data, including peer observation, charge nurse observation, and sign-in sheets. However, in practice, hand washing fell to the "honor system," with auditing by the unit charge nurse.

Results

As shown in Figure 1-2, STV's ICU VAP rate per 1,000 ventilator days decreased from the average of 8.2 per 1,000 for 13 months (January 2003–January 2004) to 3.3 per 1,000 for 24 months (February 2004–January 2006; independent 2-tailed t-test, assuming different variances, $p = .02$). The average LOS in the ICU also decreased by more than three days, from a 2003 average of 8.0 days to a January 2006 average of 4.9 days. The average number of days on a ventilator and total ventilator days also decreased.

The absence of VAPs in the ICU from the time of implementation until August 2004—a period of more than 200 days—was encouraging. Beginning in August 2004, as new VAPs were identified, each was investigated thoroughly to determine if it was due to lack of compliance with the bundle.

We celebrate each month that passes without a VAP. The MDR team is convinced the key to success in eliminating VAP is continuous staff education, keeping the concepts in front of the staff that affect the outcome, and timely reporting of the data to support the changes made.

Discussion

Data from both SJHMC and STV showed a positive impact on patient care through the implementation of the CL and VAP bundles, respectively. Both hospitals attended the IHI collaborative together and networked via conference calls as they implemented their initiatives. Each facility had a focused effort, although each facility implemented both bundles and MDR.

The implementation of the CL bundle led to a reduction of CR-BSI of more than 50% at SJHMC. The results may be an underestimate of the effect of the intervention because we included all patients in the ICU with CLs—both those for whom the bundle was implemented and those for whom it was not. The intervention is similar to that described by Render et al., who reported that adhering to maximum sterile barrier and the use of chlorhexidine antisepsis resulted in a 50%

FIGURE 1-2. St. Vincent's Hospital ICU Ventilator-Associated Pneumonia, July 2003–January 2006

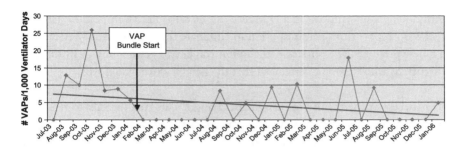

St. Vincent's Hospital intensive care unit (ICU) ventilator-associated pneumonia (VAP) rates are shown.
Source: Authors.

reduction in CR-BSI.[21] Whereas Render et al. found adherence to chlorhexidine in about 50% of the cases, we enforced the use of chlorhexidine by having it as the only antisepsis available in the CL kit, making it extremely difficult for the physician to use other antisepsis agents such as betadine. We were also able to prolong the mean time to developing a CR-BSI to up to two weeks by 2005. The compliance with CL bundle prevents early infection of CLs. Late infections are usually related to either hub contamination or progressive catheter colonization postplacement leading to CR-BSI. We are preparing educational materials that address appropriate line care.

STV, whose efforts were associated with marked reduction in VAPs, used a care bundle that included the IHI components in addition to oral care.[16,22] Unlike SJHMC, physician support at STV was minimal. In addition, the lack of presence of intensivists made it more difficult to implement the sedation vacation component of the bundle. However, the VAP rates improved significantly, and the effect of the intervention mirrored the results reported by Resar et al.[22] We believe that HOB elevation and oral care had a major impact on reducing the VAP rates.

STV found initial resistance from nursing regarding elevating the HOB, which was based on concern for the increased risk of pressure ulcers and increased risk of complications with blood pressure. Through education of the staff and physicians about the reduced risk for VAP in patients in semirecumbent positioning, especially in patients receiving enteral nutrition,[23] it was able to improve compliance.

Introducing a new process in any facility can be difficult. An important part of the success was support from administration to eliminate the barriers usually encountered with a new project.[21] The physician champion was key to getting buy-in from skeptical physicians who were not convinced that the new practice would work.

The success of the quality improvement changes were tied directly to regular use of an interdisciplinary team supported by administration with good data collection, thorough analysis, and regular reporting to reinforce the changes.[24] Monthly feedback was important because it made everyone accountable and kept these initiatives a priority. (Information was not publicly posted for families to review.)

We did not achieve all our goals. At SJHMC, the electronic database for tracking CLs did not work as intended; the system was difficult to use, and limited staffing on the IV team prevented successful implementation. In addition, checklists for some CLs that were inserted in the ICU were often missing because of the difficulty in tracking CLs. Future implementation of electronic medical records should facilitate tracking.

Successful change comes slowly and requires persistence by members of the MDR team and solid support from administration to impact culture. Flexibility on the part of unit managers, charge nurses, and staff is a primary characteristic required to affect the change process. SJHMC saw the benefit of having the physical presence of the ICPs in the ICUs, providing the staff with on-the-spot reinforcement of the initiative. STV found by starting the change process through use of a flexible MDR team, the hospital was able to successfully implement positive changes in its ICU culture. On the basis of the success in the ICU, the concept of MDR teams eventually was adapted and spread to all units in STV. Open communication among all patient caregivers was extended and served to provide improved patient care throughout the hospital.

SJHMC and STV have used a systemwide Web site to share their experiences, including educational material and tools that they developed, with other Ascension Health hospitals. In addition, prevention of nosocomial infections has been a frequent topic of monthly educational conference calls held among all the hospitals. We continue to improve our processes and share successes and barriers, thus contributing to "Healthcare That Is Safe" and to our goal of zero preventable injuries and deaths by July 2008. ■

Note: The authors thank all the health care workers who helped make this effort successful, especially Debi Hopfner (SJHMC) and Becky McKinney and Kay Como (STV).

References

1. Pryor D.B., et al.: The clinical transformation of Ascension Health: Eliminating all preventable injuries and deaths. *Jt Comm J Qual Patient Saf* 32:299–308, Jun. 2006.

2. Rose J., et al.: A leadership framework for culture change in health care. *Jt Comm J Qual Patient Saf* 32:433–442, Aug. 2006.

3. Burke J.P.: Infection control: A problem for patient safety. *N Engl J Med* 348:651–656, Feb. 13, 2003.

4. Coffin S.E., Zaoutis T.E.: Infection control, hospital epidemiology and patient safety. *Infect Dis Clin N Am* 19:647–665, Sep. 19, 2005.

5. Stone P.W., Larson E., Kawar L.N.: A systemic audit of economic evidence linking nosocomial infections and infection control interventions: 1990–2000. *Am J Infect Control* 30:145–152, May 30, 2002.

6. O'Grady N.P., et al.: The Healthcare Infection Control Practices Advisory Committee. Guidelines for the prevention of intravascular catheter-related infections. *MMWR* 51 (RR-10), Aug. 9, 2002.

7. Tablan O.C., et al.: CDC and the Healthcare Infection Control Practices Committee. Guidelines for preventing health care–associated pneumonia, 2003. *MMWR* 53 (RR-3), Mar. 26, 2004.

8. Crnich C.J., Maki D.G.: The promise of novel technology for the prevention of intravascular device–related bloodstream infection. I. Pathogenesis and short-term devices. *Clin Infect Dis* 34:1232–1242, May 1, 2002.

9. Merrer J., et al.: Complications of femoral and subclavian venous catheterization in critically ill patients: A randomized controlled trial. *JAMA* 286:700–707, Aug. 8, 2001.

10. Safdar N., Kluger D.M., Maki D.G.: A review of risk factors for catheter-related bloodstream infection caused by percutaneously inserted, noncuffed central venous catheters: Implications for preventive strategies. *Medicine* 81:466–479, Nov. 2002.

11. Kollef M.H.: Prevention of hospital-associated pneumonia and ventilator-associated pneumonia. *Crit Care Med* 32:1396–1405, Jun. 2004.

12. American Thoracic Society: Guidelines for the management of adults with hospital-acquired, ventilator-associated, and healthcare associated pneumonia. *Am J Respir Crit Care Med* 171:388–416, Feb. 15, 2005.

13. Chastre J., Fagon J.Y.: Ventilator-associated pneumonia. *Am J Respir Crit Care Med* 165:867–903, Apr. 1, 2002.

14. National Nosocomial Infections Surveillance (NNIS) System report, data summary from January 1992 to June 2004, issued October 2004. *Am J Infect Control* 30:470–485, Dec. 2004.

15. Institute for Health Care Improvement: *Implement the Central Line Bundle.* http://www.ihi.org/IHI/Topics/CriticalCare/IntensiveCare/Changes/ ImplementtheCentralLineBundle.htm (accessed Jan. 25, 2007).

16. Brunelle D.: Impact of a dedicated infusion therapy team on the reduction of catheter-related nosocomial infections, *J Infus Nurs* 26:362–365, Nov.–Dec. 2003.

17. Institute for Health Care Improvement: *Implement the Ventilator Bundle.* http://www.ihi.org/IHI/Topics/CriticalCare/IntensiveCare/Changes/ ImplementtheVentilatorBundle.htm (accessed Jan. 25, 2007).

18. Attia J., et al.: Deep vein thrombosis and its prevention in critically ill adults. *Arch Intern Med* 161:1268–1279, May 28, 2001.

19. Cook D., et al.: Risk factors for clinically important upper gastrointestinal bleeding in patients requiring mechanical ventilation, Canadian Critical Care Trials Group. *Crit Care Med* 27:2812–2817, Dec. 27, 1999.

20. Orozco-Levi M., et al.: Semirecumbent position protects from pulmonary aspiration but not completely from gastroesophageal reflux in mechanically ventilated patients. *Am J Respir Crit Care Med* 152:1387–1390, Oct. 1995.

21. Render M.L., et al.: Evidence-based practice to reduce central line infections. *Jt Comm J Qual Patient Saf* 32:253–260, May 2006.

22. Resar R., et al.: Using a bundle approach to improve ventilator care processes and reduce ventilator-associated pneumonia. *Jt Comm J Qual Patient Saf* 31:243–248, May 2005.

23. Drakulovic M.B., et al.: Supine body position as a risk factor for nosocomial pneumonia in mechanically ventilated patients: A randomized trial. *Lancet* 354:1851–1858, Nov. 27, 1999.

24. Curtis R.J., et al.: Intensive care quality improvement: A how-to guide for the interdisciplinary team. *Crit Care Med* 34:211–218, Jan. 2006.

This chapter first appeared in the November 2006 (Volume 32, Number 11, pages 612–620) issue of *The Joint Commission Journal on Quality and Patient Safety.*

A Statewide Voluntary Patient Safety Initiative: The Georgia Experience

Kimberly J. Rask, M.D., Ph.D.
Linda D. Schuessler, M.S.
Dorothy "Vi" Naylor

Voluntary reporting of medical errors and patient safety events is not new. The Institute for Safe Medication Practice (ISMP) began its Medication Error Reporting Program more than 25 years ago.[1] The confidential national program analyzes system causes of medication errors and provides recommendations for prevention. Other examples of national voluntary reporting programs include the Food and Drug Administration's MedWatch for errors related to medical products and the National Nosocomial Infections Surveillance System, sponsored by the Centers for Disease Control and Prevention.[2] Although these reporting systems are important, the Institute of Medicine (IOM) report, *To Err Is Human*, called for the development of voluntary, confidential reporting systems that are broader in scope for the primary purpose of promoting quality improvement (QI) in health care organizations.[3] Health care leaders in Georgia were focusing attention on patient safety, with the state legislature moving toward mandatory reporting requirements, even before the IOM report. In 1999, the Georgia Hospital Association (GHA) partnered with 75 stakeholder organizations in the state, including hospital systems, professional organizations, and regulatory agencies, to create a statewide voluntary patient safety program. The Partnership for Health and Accountability (PHA) was designed to be a voluntary and comprehensive patient safe-

About the Authors

Kimberly J. Rask, M.D., Ph.D., is Associate Professor of Health Policy and Management, Emory Center on Health Outcomes and Quality (ECHOQ), Atlanta, and **Linda D. Schuessler, M.S.**, formerly Project Manager, ECHOQ, is Manager, Wellness Promotion, Fiserv, Inc., Brookfield, Wisconsin.

Dorothy "Vi" Naylor is Executive Vice-President, Georgia Hospital Association, Marietta, Georgia.

Please address questions or comments to Kimberly J. Rask, krask@emory.edu.

ty program, broader than the state-mandated reporting system for sentinel events. The collaborators were able, through negotiations with policymakers, to achieve two goals that were critical in attracting broadscale participation by hospitals throughout the state. First, they established PHA as a peer review organization, ensuring the level of confidentiality necessary for free exchange of information regarding quality and medical errors. Second, a state regulatory agency approved the PHA program as meeting a state-mandated requirement that hospitals participate in a statewide patient safety program. The PHA patient safety program was built on the underlying philosophy that facilitating the ability of a diverse range of hospitals to measure, monitor, and share outcomes would translate into a safer health care system. In 2006—more than five years later—all 148 eligible Georgia hospitals are actively involved in ongoing initiatives that are part of the voluntary patient safety system. This chapter highlights the design elements that are particularly important for sustaining the initiative, along with the partnership's experience with member participation in reporting activities and patient safety improvement processes.

Creating a Sustainable Structure

Bringing together a diverse mix of hospitals in a relatively large state like Georgia is a challenge. Half the state's hospitals have fewer than 100 beds, and the state's hospital systems are evenly split between urban (54%) and rural (46%) locations. PHA could succeed only if hospitals were actively engaged in the process and able to play a significant role in guiding the direction of the initiative. For this reason, PHA was established as a peer-driven organizational structure with committees composed of representatives from each constituency, including more than 100 hospital representatives and physicians (*see* Table 2-1). (PHA provides active staff support for the committee structure by coordinating meetings and performing administrative tasks.) Each member hospital has a PHA field representative who interacts with his or her designated hospitals regularly, including site visits twice a year (*see* Table 2-2). As specialists in QI and patient safety processes, the four field representatives act as catalysts, program coordinators, and an all-around resource for PHA member hospitals, such as in informing them of best practices from other hospitals. Although actively involving members and supporting them with a hands-on approach are vital to sustaining the program, three design elements have also enhanced the program's success—leveraging existing reporting, promoting a nonpunitive environment, and using technology to facilitate communication.

TABLE 2-1. Examples of Partnership for Health and Accountability (PHA) Subcommittees*

Safe Medication Use
Members: pharmacists, nurses, physicians

- Reviews medication errors data to determine imminent and potential problems
- Identifies and promotes safe medication use system designs and practices
- Analyzes and reviews medication-related sentinel events prior to their submission to the peer review panel

Best Practices
Members: physicians, nurses, pharmacists, risk managers, QI/PI staff

- Reviews evidence-based best practices and promotes the adoption of those that are broadly accepted
- Shares aggregate data with participating hospitals and providers, and assists them in identifying opportunities for improved practices and procedures
- Guides the clinical studies, setting target thresholds for the indicators[†]

Patient Safety Issues
Members: nurses, pharmacists, risk managers, QI/PI staff, and physicians

- Designates selected patient safety areas (non–medication related) as statewide priorities
- Reviews and analyzes reports on all non–medication related sentinel events prior to submission to the PHA peer review panel

Event-Reporting Task Force
Members: risk managers, pharmacists, QI/PI staff, and nurses

- Developed online reporting tool and methodology used by health care organizations to report sentinel event information
- Evaluates and streamlines reporting requirements to avoid duplicative efforts
- Explores ways to facilitate and encourage intra- and interhospital sharing of reports to identify potential solutions

[*] QI/PI, quality improvement/performance improvement.
[†] Performed by a clinical process team within the subcommittee.

Source: Authors.

LEVERAGING EXISTING REPORTING

Given time constraints that staff at all hospitals face, PHA attempts to ensure that the voluntary reporting structure avoids redundancy with existing regulatory (for example, Centers for Medicare & Medicaid Services) and accreditation requirements (The Joint Commission) and minimizes new data collection. For example, if an event that a hospital is reporting using the PHA's online event reporting tool falls under the auspices of state-mandated reporting, the system

TABLE 2-2. Examples of Partnership for Health and Accountability (PHA) Programs That Facilitate and Support Practice Change Through Dissemination and Implementation Support

Dissemination	Implementation
Informs hospitals of prevention strategies, high-risk situations, and new guidelines via the following: • Safety alerts • E-newsletters • Other publications	PHA field representatives provide on-site technical support for improvement processes
Provides centralized, easy access via the Internet: • Evidence-based practices • Tools such as bulletin board kits	Facilitates change via local self-assessment and monitoring components through the following: • Clinical studies • Safe medication use improvement plans • Safety issue action plans • Patient safety award programs
Organizes teleconferences, conferences, or presentations on timely topics of interest	Actively involves influential local providers and administrators on committees and as leaders
Facilitates the sharing of data, best practices, and issues among hospitals	Brings together peers from across the state's medical community
Conducts orientations to new initiatives or tools	Provides administrative structure for improvement activities and reduces the burden on individual hospitals

Source: Authors.

prompts for and produces the state reporting form. The form can then be printed and faxed to the state. Both PHA and the state are notified about the event, but information identifying the hospital goes only to the state. The state regulatory agency receives the information that it needs to monitor selected events, while PHA receives more detailed information about the underlying factors that may have contributed to the event. PHA then provides a template that the reporting hospital can use to analyze underlying factors and subsequently develop an improvement plan.

PHA also uses this information to develop safety alerts, which are electronically distributed to hospitals statewide. PHA also uses statewide hospital discharge data to monitor and trend Agency for Healthcare Research and Quality (AHRQ) Inpatient Quality Indicators and Patient Safety Indicators.[4] Use of discharge data already reported to PHA entails no additional data collection efforts by hospitals.

PROMOTING A NONPUNITIVE ENVIRONMENT

A hospital staff member's willingness to come forward when a mistake occurs depends on how the organization handles blame and punishment.[5-7] PHA designed its processes to promote the adoption of open communication and a nonpunitive environment, which it recognizes as two of the pillars supporting a culture of safety. State peer-review protection laws make PHA a safe place for the open sharing of data and information, both problems and successes. Reporting becomes an opportunity for QI, with process support from PHA staff. A reported error is accompanied by an anticipated plan for improvement, which presents the opportunity for learning, even from a near miss. Hospitals benefit from others' reporting not only through learning from their experiences but also from the trending and analysis that is possible using statewide data.

USING TECHNOLOGY TO FACILITATE COMMUNICATION

Telephone conferences and the Internet allow geographically diverse hospitals to participate fully in PHA programs and committees, to access tools and information, and to keep abreast of patient safety issues and best practices. PHA's Web site (http://www.gha.org/pha) contains both public areas and a proprietary (password-protected) section, which is a source for information on QI initiatives and best practices; a calendar of meetings, events, and deadlines; and resources and toolkits. The proprietary section also enables access to the online event reporting system. PHA holds many of its committee meetings via teleconference, coordinates educational teleconferences, publishes a weekly e-newsletter, and sends out periodic safety alerts when an issue warrants prompt attention.

Participation and Outcomes

The best gauge of success for a voluntary reporting system is typically the level of participation.

REPORTING TO THE LAY PUBLIC

PHA publishes an annual statewide hospital-specific report, *Insights*,[8] which is available to the public. This report tracks individual hospital participation in voluntary clinical improvement initiatives, such as Collaborative QI Partnerships, as well as their performance on Joint Commission core measures. Hospitals decide whether they want their outcomes published. For each indicator, performance is noted in terms of whether the hospital scored in the top 10% or top 50% for Joint Commission–accredited hospitals. By the 2004 edition of *Insights*, 88% of hospitals included their data for Joint Commission core measures, even when their scores did not fall in the top 50%. For *Insights 2006*, 97% (144) of 148 hospitals were publicly reporting their data.[8]

PATIENT SAFETY IMPROVEMENT PROGRAMS

Hospitals have engaged in programs such as Safe Medication Use (SMU) and Patient Safety Issues–Medical Events projects. Teams composed of QI staff, physicians, and front-line employees, work together to improve clinical practices and provide safer care. PHA provides guidance and support for the projects, sets monitoring expectations, and tracks progress.

SMU. SMU is a comprehensive medication error reduction program that provides hospitals with a template and structure for analyzing internal data around medication errors and developing an improvement plan. Of 148 acute-stay member hospitals, 144 (97.3%) are now participating in this program on a voluntary basis. For improvement plans begun in 2002 or 2003, 69.1% of participating hospitals were successful in reducing the incidence of targeted errors. The mean reduction in targeted errors after nine months of follow-up was 34% in 2004.[9] Just as important, and providing evidence of their comfort with data sharing, one fifth of hospitals reported that the incidence of the targeted error had not changed or had actually increased. Hospitals with negative results were willing to report them and share their assessments of where the improvement process fell short. Small or rural hospitals were as likely as their larger or urban counterparts to see successful reductions. The most significant predictor of successful reductions in targeted errors was active participation in the PHA program, as measured by hospital staff participation in educational sessions and membership on standing committees.[9] In 2005, PHA replaced the medication error assessment tool with the ISMP self-assessment tool,[10] which enables hospitals to benchmark on a national basis. Statewide participation continues to exceed 90%, and fewer hospitals (7%) are reporting difficulty measuring outcomes.

Patient Safety Issues–Medical Events Program. This program focuses on clinical patient safety issues identified by member-driven PHA committees as having the most promise for improvement. The safety issues chosen for emphasis in 2004—deep vein thrombosis, pressure ulcers, and fall prevention—continue to be the most frequently chosen topics. Although most of the hospitals (62%) chose to participate in one of these structured improvement programs, others participated in a collaborative failure mode and effects analysis (FMEA) (12%) or designed individualized programs to target hospital-specific problem areas (14%).

Making Safety Work in the Hospital Setting

The Quality and Patient Safety Awards program creates local initiatives designed to reduce the risk of medical errors and improve patient safety and outcomes. Hospital teams from across the state vie for the awards, which are presented at the annual Patient Safety Summit. Case studies are provided below for two award-winning hospital systems—Athens Regional Hospital (out of 50 large hospital [300+ beds] system applicants) and Habersham County Medical Center (out of 31 small hospital [< 100 beds] systems).

CASE STUDY 1. ATHENS REGIONAL MEDICAL CENTER (ARMC)

With 315 beds and approximately 2,000 employees, ARMC (http://www.armc.org), is a full-service medical facility. Committed to broad-based, interdisciplinary involvement in self-assessment and improvement, ARMC involved all levels of the organization in the patient safety initiative. The hospital's SafeCare Committee, composed of medical staff leaders, nursing, pharmacy, administration, quality, risk management, and ancillary areas such as radiology, spearheaded a hospitalwide error reduction initiative in 2001. On the basis of a review of research and best practices in both health care and other industries, ARMC leaders determined that the following three factors would be key to eliminating latent and preventable errors that produce harm:

1. Providers should see health care delivery as a system of care rather than independent care tasks.

2. Methods must be developed to identify both the active and latent performance attributes that contribute to harm and are preventable.

3. The organization's culture must change in a manner that addresses the pervasive tendency to assign blame rather than seek solutions. The team analyzed available data, including those from PHA and The Joint Commission's Sentinel Event Database,[11] categorizing most preventable errors that lead to harm into three categories: omission, identification, and communication. The search for a way to analyze care delivery processes for sources of both latent and active harm led ARMC to develop the Systematic Assessment of Flow and Error (SAFE) tool (*see* Figure 2-1), for which it was recognized with a PHA award in 2003. The SAFE tool, which can be used by anyone in the organization, distills the complex, interdependent processes of health care into four main components: *patient information*, which is used to guide *clinical decisions*, which lead to *care processes*, which determine *patient flow* through the health care system. This framework was useful for promoting a systems perspective, encouraging reporting, and reducing perceptions of blame. The instrument incorporates many of The Joint Commission's National Patient Safety Goals and appears compatible with The Joint Commission's tracer methodology.[12]

The process is iterative: Information supports decisions that spawn care processes that drive patient flow. When the system flows properly, information is readily available for decisions, the time between clinical decisions is kept to a minimum, care processes proceed quickly and efficiently, and the movement of the patient is managed well and safely. Staff throughout ARMC were introduced to the use of the SAFE tool and principles of patient safety through orientations, educational sessions, and a full-day workshop. The tool removes the issue of "individual competence," promotes system thinking, and supports a nonpunitive environment that encourages reporting. As reported to staff, when the SAFE tool was used in 2002 to analyze variances, root cause analyses, and case studies, only 2.1% of errors were attributed to an individual's competence. Showing that the overwhelming majority of errors are system-related helped reduce barriers to incident reporting.

The number of staff-reported errors increased from 421 in 2002 to 542 in 2003, with the largest jump (82%) seen in errors of omission. Given this early success, the SAFE tool was subsequently used to support many patient safety initiatives at

**FIGURE 2-1. Systematic Assessment of Flow and Error (SAFE) Tool:
A System of Care**

Information - Decisions - Care Process - Patient Flow

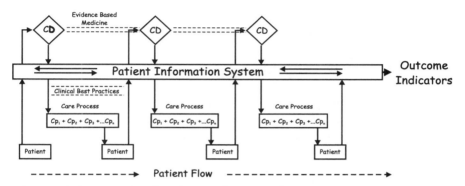

Outcome Indicators: Mortality, LOS, Readmission, Infection
Clinical Process Measures: Clinical Practice Standards
Operations Process Measures: Setup, Queue, Delay, Bottleneck, Process Time

The SAFE tool can also be used as a template for any process evaluations. For example, consider a patient presenting to the emergency room with chest pain. The initial history and assessment (patient information) leads to a clinical decision (CD), perhaps a request for lab studies and an electrocardiogram (EKG). That decision spawns a care process (draw blood, perform EKG). Information from that care process is then available for the next clinical decision (lab results, EKG results). The patient either "flows" to a new setting or other care providers "flow" to the patient. The process is iterative: Information supports decisions that spawn care processes that drive patient flow.
Source: Authors.

ARMC, including reducing laboratory turnaround times, decreasing error rates for insulin sliding scales, minimizing patient misidentification, and reducing preventable falls. For example, the diabetes improvement team found that (1) a significant number of patients experienced blood glucose levels outside desired therapeutic range during their hospital stay and (2) 37 different sliding scales were being used for calculation of insulin doses, contributing to variability in dose calculation and opportunity for error. The team developed a preprinted sliding scale order form that reduced the number of scales to 3, decreased illegibility issues, eliminated opportunities for miscalculations, and reduced ambiguity. In 2004, six months after

33

institution of the new forms and processes, chart reviews showed that the new slid-ing scale order form was used for half of all patients on sliding scales for subcuta-neous regular insulin. The total percentage of insulin dose errors decreased from 5.29% to 4.72%, while the percentage of wrong dose errors decreased from 1.95% to 0.59%. In 2005, the SAFE tool was used to address patient identification and matching for laboratory studies. The laboratory improvement team used the Six Sigma improvement model and FMEA to increase the accuracy of patient identifi-cation and matching from 75% to 96% and to improve the timeliness of laboratory results by 40%. ARMC staff continue to find benefit in sharing performance infor-mation with other health care systems in the state and particularly in participating in work sessions, where they can learn from other hospitals' successes in specific areas, such as reducing time to first-dose antibiotic for patients with pneumonia.

CASE STUDY 2. HABERSHAM COUNTY MEDICAL CENTER (HCMC)

HCMC (http://www.hcmcmed.org), has proven that a small, rural primary care hospital can make significant strides in improving patient safety. The medical center, located in northeastern Georgia, serves the surrounding area with a 53-bed acute-care facility and an 83-bed long term care facility. The HCMC Hospital Authority Board (Hospital Authority), which assumes responsibility for the quality and safety of patient care at the medical center, endorsed the PHA initiative and built the program into its Plan for Organizational Performance. The Quality Leadership Steering Committee, a physician-directed, interdiscipli-nary group, provides oversight for continuous QI activities within the medical center and reports to the Hospital Authority. In early summer 2004, the commit-tee, with assistance from PHA, the Georgia Quality Improvement Organization, and a statewide collaborative of hospitals, identified surgical infections as a target for their patient safety efforts. HCMC benchmarked its performance on surgical infections with data collected through the collaborative. The hospital subsequently broadened its focus, setting a goal to improve the overall care of and streamline processes for surgical patients. The resulting patient safety initiative, which was honored at the PHA 2004 Patient Safety Summit, was placed under the supervi-sion of a newly chartered postoperative care team that oversaw several focused care improvement teams. The care improvement teams were composed of man-agers, administrators, and care providers, with 11 departments represented. The teams met monthly for the first 18 months to identify barriers, monitor outcomes,

FIGURE 2-2. Postoperative Pneumonia Rates at Habersham County Medical Center, 2004–2005

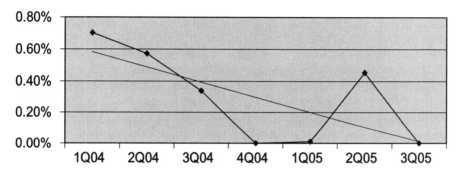

Results since 2004 include a decrease of more than 50% in the postoperative pneumonia rate and a 0% surgical infection rate in the pilot population of 172 inpatient orthopedic cases for the first 12 months.

Source: Authors.

and develop solutions. Several new programs were implemented, including a pulmonary management and pneumonia prevention protocol; staff and patient/family education; a preoperative physical therapy evaluation; and timely notification to physical therapy, case management, and home care to allow comprehensive discharge planning. Results since 2004 include a decrease of more than 50% in the postoperative pneumonia rate and a 0% surgical infection rate in the pilot population of 172 inpatient orthopedic cases for the first 12 months (*see* Figure 2-2). Like ARMC, HCMC has found it valuable to network with other providers and work collaboratively to identify initiatives that improve patient outcomes.

Discussion

Creating and maintaining a voluntary patient safety system presents major challenges and depends on key factors (*see* Table 2-3). Although there have been successes and encouraging signs that hospital systems in the state are engaged in the process, there are important caveats.

Table 2-3. Factors Key to Partnership for Health and Accountability

- **Trust.** Previous shared experiences and a confidential environment foster an atmosphere of trust.
- **Stability.** Long-standing relationships instill confidence in its viability and longevity.
- **Grassroots involvement.** Involving committed staff leaders facilitates buy-in at the local level.
- **Local ownership.** Empowering local teams to address their unique issues enhances learning and creates a sense of ownership.
- **Tailoring.** Flexibility allows productive participation across diverse hospitals.
- **Dovetailing.** The burden on hospitals is minimized by building on existing programs and initiatives.
- **Communication.** Teleconference and Internet communication channels are leveraged.
- **Perspective.** The issues facing hospitals are monitored.
- **Iterative process.** The nonpunitive environment supports a continuous cycle of evaluation, development, and execution of action plans.

Source: Authors.

CREATING A STRONG YET FLEXIBLE UMBRELLA ORGANIZATION

A voluntary patient safety initiative should not be confused with a system that is led by volunteers or representatives from collaborating organizations that take time from their normal responsibilities to administer the program. From the beginning, the GHA allocated resources in the form of paid staff that initially were dedicated to building the PHA initiative, and AHRQ supplied partial funding for three subsequent years to help jump-start the program and support a multidimensional evaluation of program outcomes. Since the completion of the AHRQ funding, the GHA Board has continued funding the program. At the same time, however, PHA staff had to resist "taking over." It was essential that there be a sense of local ownership and involvement at all levels of the hospital organization because the program's success is ultimately dependent on local adoption and implementation. It was also critical that PHA staff remain flexible and willing to listen to the concerns and suggestions of hospital administrators, physicians, and staff while still maintaining the integrity of the patient safety efforts.

Streamlining Data Collection

A voluntary program's long-term success is also critically dependent on the design of data collection and reporting systems that minimize the administrative burden for hospitals. Although PHA built its programs on the framework of existing reporting requirements and assessment structures, hospitals soon voiced resistance for "extra" paperwork that PHA required. Working with peer-driven committees, PHA reduced the frequency of reporting and, as described, developed a new Web tool to eliminate duplication of event reporting. Streamlining of reporting processes is evaluated at least yearly, and at the request of the member hospitals, PHA continually reevaluates data collection tools to provide better data feedback and education while still minimizing duplicative efforts.

TRUSTING THE ITERATIVE PROCESS

Achieving significant organizational change is complex. Because of competing internal and external forces, systemic change requires a long-term focus. PHA has learned that building clinical, cultural, and system improvements for safe patient care involves an iterative process, requiring patience and persistence. Typically, for example, hospitals have required three cycles of process improvement plans, incorporating feedback, to show positive results. With experience, hospitals are able to better identify the key stakeholders, data, and processes necessary to ensure success.

NEXT STEPS

PHA continues to evolve, adding new programs, as described below, while streamlining previous data requirements for its members. As more resources for patient safety improvement programs become available from federal agencies and nonprofit organizations, PHA is incorporating these processes to avoid duplication and concentrate its efforts where there are gaps or where a customized approach is desirable. Building on the last five years of initiatives, PHA is positioned to become a Patient Safety Organization, as created by federal legislation.[13] PHA is also continuing efforts to expand its Web site, create toolkits, develop collaboratives for high-priority patient safety issues, and provide educational resources for programs such as rapid response teams, medication reconciliation, and the GHA Patient Safety Improvement Corps program, an AHRQ–supported initiative modeled after the AHRQ and Veterans Health Administration National Patient Safety Improvement Corps training program.[14] PHA and hospital quality staff participated in this year-long national program in 2004–2005, which was conducted through workshops, site visits, and telephone conferences. Another natural progression for PHA's patient safety initiatives is the development of a Hospital Relative Quality Index (HRQI). The HRQI provides PHA with a method to compare hospitals across process, outcomes, and medication safety. Because the GHA maintains the only statewide database of hospital process, discharge, and patient safety data, a quality index can be created without requiring additional work or effort by hospitals. The HRQI not only translates data into information that hospitals can use to improve quality and customer satisfaction but it is a user-friendly report to help consumers make better-informed health care decisions. The HRQI score is included in *Insights 2006*[8] and is publicly distributed.

Although these are positive steps toward the goal of establishing a self-sustaining QI program, the challenge for PHA will be to maintain a program that is relevant, stable, and integrated and meets the needs of a diverse group of hospitals and yet remains flexible enough to evolve as systems and patient safety priorities change. ■

Note: The project described in this chapter was supported by Grant Number 1 U18 HS11918 from the Agency for Healthcare Research and Quality (AHRQ). The content of this chapter does not necessarily reflect the views or policies of AHRQ. The authors assume full responsibility for the accuracy and completeness of the ideas presented. The authors acknowledge the staff and hospital liaisons for the Partnership for Health and Accountability and thank them for their support in developing this chapter. They specifically acknowledge Janice McKenzie and Jane Anderson (Habersham County Medical Center) and Steve Mayfield (formerly at Athens Regional Medical Center and currently executive director, Quality Center, American Hospital Association), for their assistance with the case studies.

References

1. Institute for Safe Medication Practices: *USP-ISMP Medication Errors Reporting Program (MERP)*. https://www.ismp.org/orderForms/reporterrortoISMP.asp (accessed Jan. 24, 2007).

2. Agency for Healthcare Research and Quality: *Patient Safety Reporting Systems and Research in HHS*. http://www.ahrq.gov/qual/taskforce/hhsrepor.htm (accessed Jan. 24, 2007).

3. Institute of Medicine: *To Err Is Human: Building a Safer Health System*. Washington, DC: National Academy Press, 1999.

4. Agency for Healthcare Research and Quality (AHRQ): *AHRQ Quality Indicators*. http://www.qualityindicators.ahrq.gov/ (accessed Jan. 24, 2007).

5. Beyea S.C.: Creating a just safety culture. AORN 79:412–414, Feb. 2004.

6. Marx D.: *Patient Safety and the "Just Culture": A Primer for Health Care Executives*. New York: Columbia University Press, 2001.

7. Ruchlin H.S., et al.: The role of leadership in instilling a culture of safety: Lessons from the literature. *J Healthcare Manag* 49:47–48, Jan.–Feb. 2004.

8. Partnership for Health and Accountability: *Insights* 2006. http://www.gha.org/pha/Insights/2006/index.asp (accessed Jan. 25, 2007).

9. Rask K.J., et al.: Impact of a statewide reporting system on medication error reduction. *J Patient Safety*, in press.

10. Institute for Safe Medication Practices (ISMP): *ISMP Self-Assessments*. http://www.ismp.org/selfassessments/default.asp (accessed Jan. 25, 2007).

11. The Joint Commission: *Sentinel Event Statistics–June 30, 2006*. http://www.jointcommission.org/SentinelEvents/Statistics/ (accessed Jan. 24, 2007).

12. Joint Commission Resources: Continuous Survey Readiness Workshop, Summer Update. Macon, GA, Jul. 31–Aug. 1, 2003.

13. Agency for Healthcare Research and Quality: *The Patient Safety and Quality Improvement Act of 2005*. Overview, Jun. 2006. http://www.ahrq.gov/qual/psoact.htm (accessed Jan. 25, 2007).

14. Agency for Healthcare Research and Quality (AHRQ): *Patient Safety Improvement Corps: An AHRQ/VA Partnership*. May 2005. http://www.ahrq.gov/about/psimpcorps.htm (accessed Jan. 25, 2007).

This chapter first appeared in the October 2006 (Volume 32, Number 10, pages 564–572) issue of *The Joint Commission Journal on Quality and Patient Safety*.

Using Real-Time Problem Solving to Eliminate Central Line Infections

Richard P. Shannon, M.D.

Diane Frndak, M.B.A., P.A.-C.

Naida Grunden

Jon C. Lloyd, M.D.

Cheryl Herbert, R.N.

Bhavin Patel, M.D.

Daniel Cummins

Alexander H. Shannon

Paul H. O'Neill

Steven J. Spear, D.B.A.

Central line–associated bloodstream infections (CLABs) exact a tremendous human cost. Of approximately 4 million patients admitted to intensive care units (ICUs) in the United States each year,[1] 48% receive indwelling central catheters to ease the delivery of medication and/or nutrition.[2] That translates to 15 million central catheter days.[3–5] Approximately 200,000 patients contract bloodstream infections from these catheters each year. These infections, which are often considered the inevitable collateral damage that accompanies complex critical care, come with associated mortality of 15% to 20%.[3–6] The financial costs are also considerable, with estimates of $3,700 to $29,000 per infection.[5]

Despite knowledge of the guidelines on central line placement developed by the Centers for Disease Control and

About the Authors

Richard P. Shannon, M.D., is the Claude R. Joyner Professor of Medicine, Drexel University College of Medicine, and Chairman, Department of Medicine, Allegheny General Hospital, Pittsburgh.

Diane Frndak M.B.A., P.A.-C., is Director of Quality Performance, West Penn-Allegheny Health System, Pittsburgh.

Naida Grunden is Communications Director, Pittsburgh Regional Healthcare Initiative, Pittsburgh.

Jon C. Lloyd, M.D., is Regional MRSA Prevention Coordinator, Centers for Disease Control and Prevention, VA Pittsburgh Health System, Pittsburgh.

Cheryl Herbert, R.N., is Director, Infection Control, Allegheny General Hospital.

Bhavin Patel, M.D., was a third-year medical resident, and **Daniel Cunnins** and **Alexander H. Shannon** were summer interns, Department of Medicine, Allegheny General Hospital.

Hon. Paul H. O'Neill, the former Secretary of the Treasury, is a founding member of the Pittsburgh Regional Healthcare Initiative.

Steven J. Spear, D.B.A., is a Senior Director, Institute for Healthcare Improvement, Cambridge, Massachusetts.

Please address reprint requests to Richard P. Shannon, M.D., rshannon@wpahs.org.

Prevention (CDC),[7] in 2002 Allegheny General Hospital (AGH) reported an average of 5.1 infections per 1,000 line days in its medical intensive care (MICU) and coronary care units (CCU). This rate was somewhat better than the National Nosocomial Infection System (NNIS) average for comparable units (5.4 per 1,000 line-days).[8]

Questioning whether this complication rate was acceptable, in April 2003, the chairman of the department of medicine [R.S.], in collaboration with ICU staff and in partnership with the Pittsburgh Regional Healthcare Institute (PRHI), set the goal of eliminating them. AGH looked for methods to improve performance and discovered powerful examples within industry. They found that a few organizations, such as Toyota and Alcoa, have superior internal operations. Even though they provide similar products and services to similar markets as their competitors and use similar process technology, they achieve superior levels of quality, productivity, efficiency, flexibility, and safety. This level of performance is sustained through superior rates of improvement across broad ranges of products, processes, and functions.[9,10]

Leaders' improvement abilities lie in how they manage work to reveal problems as they occur and solve problems as they are revealed. Whereas many health care organizations try to solve problems with retrospective analysis of aggregated data, high-performing organizations improve their work at the time and place where inefficiencies, difficulties, and errors occur.[11–17] Doing so allows problems to be solved in context, taking advantage of information that is tacit to the interaction and that would be lost if aggregated or reported retrospectively.[18–20] The result is a continuous building of process knowledge and performance improvement.

The study reported in this article was designed to determine whether (1) the application of process improvement techniques used by Toyota could be applied to the rapid elimination of central line infections in two ICUs and (2) the results were sustainable during a three-year period. This article represents a more complete and up-to-date treatment of the ideas introduced elsewhere.[21] Reduction of CLABs was subsequently included as a plank in the Institute for Healthcare Improvement's 100,000 Lives Campaign. The campaign recently reported that it has exceeded its expectation with an estimated 122,300 lives saved.[22] AGH served as a mentor hospital for the campaign.

Methods

SETTING

AGH is a 778-bed academic health center serving Pittsburgh and the surrounding three-state area. The hospital annually admits nearly 32,000 patients and employs 4,600 people, including approximately 1,250 physicians. AGH is a major teaching affiliate of the Drexel University College of Medicine. The work was focused in the MICU and CCU, which comprised 28 contiguous beds with more than 1,700 admissions a year. Twenty-one critical care fellows and 60 internal medicine residents, as well as third- and fourth-year students, rotate through the MICU and CCU. Because this study was part of a quality improvement (QI) effort, an Institutional Review Board waiver was obtained.

PERFECTING PATIENT CARE™

The AGH working group drew on a local community resource, the Pittsburgh Regional Health Initiative (PRHI)[23,24] to learn about process improvement techniques rooted in the Toyota Production System (Lean thinking). AGH physicians, nurses, and infection control practitioners received five days of intensive training at PRHI in the improvement system called Perfecting Patient Care (PPC)[21,23-25] and then applied those principles in clinical practice. The team, headed by the chairman of the department of medicine, also included unit directors, infection control nurses, ICU nurses, and staff from PRHI [D.F., N.G., J.C.L.].

The PPC methods used at AGH entailed the following five steps:

1. Establish the true dimension of the current problem and establish zero as the goal.
2. Observe the actual work to find opportunities to standardize processes and stabilize systems.
3. Move quickly from retrospective data to actionable, real-time data analyzed and acted on immediately with every symptomatic patient.
4. Solve problems one by one as close to the time and place of occurrence as possible.
5. Provide continuous education in both process improvement and technique for new and rotating staff members.

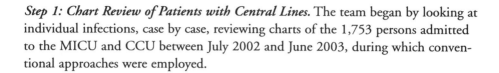

Step 1: Chart Review of Patients with Central Lines. The team began by looking at individual infections, case by case, reviewing charts of the 1,753 persons admitted to the MICU and CCU between July 2002 and June 2003, during which conventional approaches were employed.

Step 2: Observation of Line Placement and Maintenance. With a clearer sense of the frequency, types, and consequences of CLABs in its MICU and CCU, the team began observing staff to determine how lines were actually placed and maintained. Ten residents, 10 fellows, 8 attending physicians, 16 nurses, 6 nurse's aides, and 5 personnel responsible for providing materials were directly observed as they worked. A total of 40 hours of observations were conducted involving 8 central line placements and 12 line maintenance procedures. These observations revealed material, method, training, communication, and other subtle factors that compromised line placement and maintenance.

Step 3: Real-Time Investigation of Individual Infections. At the same time that AGH's team studied and improved placement and maintenance methods, it searched for other possible causes by investigating any CLABs as soon as they were identified. Infections were initially defined as CLABs if they met one of three CDC criteria.[8]

During the period from July 2003 through June 2004, all positive blood cultures were reported to the infection control nurse [C.H.], who quickly investigated and classified them according to admitting diagnosis, origin, infection site, line duration before infection, and in-hospital mortality. Each occurrence was examined to its root cause as close as possible to receipt of a positive lab culture (range, 3–24 hours; average, 6 hours, including weekends). The root cause team investigating each occurrence included the infection control nurse, the physician of record, and the residents, fellows, and nurses caring for the patient. The team was headed by the chairman of the department of medicine.

Step 4: Developing Countermeasures. The results of the observations and real-time problem solving were new processes and procedures, collaboratively developed, which began as stopgaps or "countermeasures" (*see* Results). Four major countermeasures were developed and adopted in the first 90 days, but each new CLAB occurrence created new opportunities for learning and improving processes.

Step 5: Continuous Learning. Solving problems in real time allowed the team to determine that training in central line placement was inadequate. The team developed a countermeasure that required new trainees (nurses and physicians) to be educated in a multidisciplinary training exercise using patient simulators with the guidance of physician mentors and nursing staff. Multidisciplinary training allowed all team members to understand the work standardization and their specific roles in an unambiguous way. Residents and fellows were also reeducated in subclavian line placement technique, and a portable ultrasound machine was provided to facilitate vein localization. Antimicrobial dressings were used for all catheters remaining in place for longer than seven days and on all femoral catheters inserted emergently.

MEASUREMENTS AND ANALYTIC METHODS

We compared the number of CLABs and mortality associated with them before (fiscal year [FY] 03) and after (FY04–FY06) the initiation of the PPC approach. We expressed the improvement in simple unambiguous terms such as number of patients infected and the risk of infection associated with a central line. We also expressed the improvement in process reliability as the risk of infections, defined as the number of infections per number of lines placed.

Clinical outcomes were compared using the chi-square test (age, sex, frequency, rates, lines) and Fisher's exact test (mortality, reliability). Differences were considered statistically significant if the $p < .05$.

Results

Between July 2002 and June 2003, the reported rate of CLABS, on the basis of NNIS criteria, in the MICU and CCU was 5.1 infections/1,000 line-days. When these data were decoded and reported in clinical terms, a dramatically different picture emerged (*see* Table 3-1). Of the 37 patients who had a CLAB, up to one third suffered more than one infection (total CLABs, 49). Nineteen (51%) of the 37 patients died in the hospital. The unadjusted mortality rate of patients with CLABs was twice the overall mortality rate in the two ICUs (21%). Even when compared with critically ill, ventilated patients (35% mortality), patients with CLABs had a one- to twofold greater mortality.

The microbiology of CLABs involved more virulent organisms (*Staphylococcus aureus*, methicillin-resistant *Staphylococcus aureus*, and Gram-negative rods) likely contributing to the excess mortality. Importantly, femoral catheters accounted for

TABLE 3-1. Summary of Findings from Chart Review, Medical Intensive Care Unit and Coronary Care Unit, July 2002–June 2003*

Number of patients	1,753
Number of patients with central lines	1,067
Number of patients with central line–associated bloodstream infections	37
Number of central line–associated bloodstream infections	49
Infection Sites	
Femoral	21
Internal jugular	14
Subclavian	8
Radial arterial	3
Percutaneous (PICC)	3
Infections/1,000 line-days	10.5
Total Number of Lines Employed	193
Lines/patient	5.2
In-hospital mortality of central line–associated bloodstream infection patients	19 of 37 (51%)
Unit's overall in-hospital mortality	368 of 1,753 (21%)
In-hospital mortality of patients with DRG 475[†]	52/153 (35%)
Average Duration of Line Before Infections (days)	
Femoral	6 (2–9)
Internal jugular	8 (4–13)
Subclavian	14 (10–28)
Radial arterial	6 (4–8)
Percutaneous (PICC)	17 (8–32)
Organisms	
Coagulase-negative *Staphylococcus*	17 (35%)
Staphylococcus aureus	15 (30%)
MRSA	10
Candida species	9 (19%)
Gram-negative rods	8 (16%)
* PICC, peripherally inserted central catheter; MRSA, methicillin-resistant *Staphylococcus aureus*. [†] Diagnosis-related group (DRG) 475 is used for ventilated patients with respiratory failure. This was the most common admitting diagnosis for patients who developed central line–associated bloodstream infections.	

Source: Authors.

43% of the CLABs but were not included in the NNIS definition. Therefore, they were not "counted" previously, so rates were underreported. With femoral lines included, the actual infection rate was 10.5/1,000 line-days. Thus, the magnitude of the problem was far greater in terms of the frequency of infections, the virulence of the organism, and the associated mortality than was conveyed in the epidemiological metric.

Observations revealed variations in line placement and management practices (*see* Table 3-2). Interpretations varied among nurses as to what constituted appropriate technique. For example, site selection was based on clinician preference or perceived skill in performing a certain approach. Physicians did not always explain to patients and family members the procedure's risks, benefits, and indications. Communication among team members was inconsistent, with nurses hesitant to question physicians about breaches in sterile technique or the lack of procedure notes. Often, team members did not recognize that a patient had a central line or question its continued need. Certain clinical situations lacked clear procedures. For example, should a line present on transfer from another facility be removed when its integrity could not be verified, or should it remain pending signs of induration or erythema?

On the basis of observations made by and of staff, the units developed standards for evaluating site integrity and dressing changes. Practices were standardized by adopting a single common line insertion kit, specified sterile techniques, and standardized documentation for each procedure. Line placement protocols were reviewed and implemented through unit medical directors, fellows, and house staff. The decline in femoral catheter use led to a decline in the time required to change dressings from 15 minutes to 5 minutes. The presentation of data on standardized, unambiguous bedside displays about line sites and duration eliminated time wasted by physicians looking for information. The standardized practices allowed variations to be easily identified, so their consequences could be contained before they propagated into an infection. The standardized practices were accompanied by reinforcement of the value, as expressed in weekly working sessions, that safety and reliability in line placement and maintenance were not merely a priority but a precondition to the work.

At the same time that AGH's team studied and improved placement and maintenance methods, it searched for other possible causes by investigating any CLABs as soon as they were identified. These investigations uncovered other factors that

TABLE 3-2. Observed Variations in the Practice of Central Line Placement and Care and Summary of Countermeasures that Were Developed During Step 2

Placement	
Observed sources of variation	**Resulting changes in practice**
No standard pre-procedure checklist	Pre-procedure checklist developed, including request for informed consent
Informed consent obtained infrequently (< 25%)	
No standard site specification	Standardized line insertion kit developed, including disinfectant, drape, gown, and gloves; system improvements ensure kit always available when/where needed
No standard line kit	
No standard procedure for disinfecting site prior to line placement	
No standard procedure for draping the patient	
No standard procedure for gowning and gloving	
No standard documentation of the procedure	Standardized documentation of procedure developed, implemented
Line Care	
Observed sources of variation	**Resulting changes in practice**
No standard kit for dressing lines	Standardized dressing kit developed, always available
No standard definitions for site induration	Standardized definition for erythema and induration
No standard use of disinfectant	Chlorhexidine standard as disinfectant
No standard procedure for when a dressing would be changed	Daily observation of dressing site; document dressing changes at least every 5 days
No mechanism for following line location and duration	

Source: Authors.

had not been accounted for in line placement and maintenance guidelines that AGH had developed so far. Investigating close in time and place to the actual occurrence provided contextual information that would otherwise have been lost.

For example, one patient who developed an infection had a femoral line in place for four days. Yet CDC guidelines state a preference for the subclavian site. The team investigated this site choice by asking a series of "whys," designed to reveal the root cause of the problem:

1. *Why did the patient have a femoral line?* Because the line was inserted emergently at night.
2. *Why would inserting the line at night cause a physician to choose femoral placement?* At a teaching hospital, fellows generally end their shift at 6 P.M., although several remain on call. House officers either must call a fellow in from home or insert the line themselves.
3. *Why would house officers choose the femoral site?* Because femoral lines were perceived to be easier and safer to insert than subclavian lines, on which many house officers may not yet be trained.
4. *Why would a femoral line be left in place for four days?* Because the risk of infection had been understated, there was little sense of urgency about removing that line and inserting a new one at a preferred site.

The real-time investigation and problem solving transformed central line infections from mysterious processes shrouded in inevitability to recognized processes that could be improved and error avoided. Examples of countermeasures developed using real-time problem solving included the following:

1. Remove femoral lines within 12 hours and replace with a line at a preferred site.
2. Replace dysfunctional catheters: do not rewire them.
3. Replace lines present on transfer.
4. Prefer the subclavian position for central lines.

These countermeasures were developed, implemented, and disseminated within 90 days of initiating the process. Notably, many of these countermeasures are not captured in CDC guidelines but are specific to the work and context of these ICUs.

The system redesign also included the creation of a help chain that cut through the organization's hierarchy. A nurse who experienced or observed a problem was to notify the charge nurse, who, if help was needed, would contact the unit director. Notification would continue up the help chain as necessary to the chair of medicine until the defect was addressed.

Table 3-3 illustrates the magnitude of the impact of these system redesigns on clinical outcomes. From July 2003 through June 2004 (FY04), 6 CLABs in six patients were reported in the two units, compared with 49 infections the previous year (FY03). Central line infection rates fell from 10.5 infections to 1.2 infections/1,000 line-days. In keeping with the approach of analyzing problems when they occur, all 6 infections were investigated when they were detected. Four infections involved peripherally inserted central catheter lines, 1 a subclavian line, 1 an internal jugular line. Each line was in place for more than 15 days, requiring new countermeasures to deal with chronic indwelling catheters.

As the infection rate declined, so did the associated mortality rates. In the baseline year, 19 of the 37 (51%) patients who contracted CLABs died. In the following year, the number was 1 out of 6 (17%). All 6 CLABs in FY04 were attributable to coagulase-negative staphylococcal species. Methicillin-resistant *Staphylococcus aureus*, Gram-negative organisms, and fungal infections, which had constituted two thirds of previous CLABs, were eliminated. The process reliability from 1 infection in every 22 lines placed to 1 in 185 lines placed.

Table 3-3 also illustrates the results in the second year of the continuous learning process on the basis of real-time problem solving. Notably, the number of CLABs increased from 6 to 11 patients but remained significantly lower than the incidence before the introduction of the PPC initiative. Whereas Admission Severity Group score, age, and sex distribution were not different, there was a 34% increase in line usage and a 33% increase in line-days compared with the first year of the initiative. The rate of CLAB infections was 1.6 compared with 1.2 infections/1,000 line-days, but the process reliability decreased from 1 infection in 185 lines placed to 1 infection in 135 lines placed. The associated mortality remained the same and significantly lower than that observed before the PPC initiative. Rather than view the increase in CLABs as a failure, the team applied the same principles that led to the early success and seized the opportunity to learn from these more complex cases.

TABLE 3-3. Comparison of Clinical Outcomes: Traditional Approach Versus Perfecting Patient Care (PPC) Approach*

	Traditional Approach FY 2003	PPC Approach FY 2004 Year 1	PPC Approach FY 2005 Year 2	PPC Approach FY 2006 (10 months) Year 3
Intensive care unit admissions (n)	1,753	1,798	1,829	1,832
Atlas severity grade	1.9	2.0	2.1	2.2
Age (years)	62 (24–80)	62 (50–74)	65 (39–71)	64 (52–79)
Sex (M/F)	22/15	3/3	4/7	1/2
Central lines employed (n)	1,110	1,321*	1,487*	1,898*
Line-days	4,687	5,052*	6,705*	7,716*
Infections	49	6*	11*	3*
Patients infected	37	6*	11*	3*
Rates (infections/ 1,000 line-days)	10.5	1.2*	1.6*	0.39*
Deaths	19 (51%)	1 (16%)*	2 (18%)*	0 (0%)*
Reliability (no. of lines placed to get one infection)	22	185*	135*	633*

* $p < .05$ compared with the traditional approach.

Source: Authors.

They discovered that 7 of the 11 CLABs in FY05 were in peripherally inserted central catheter (PICC) lines, where standardized processes had not been developed.

Specific and unique problems were identified with the use of PICC, including more frequent catheter manipulation and their use for phlebotomy in addition to infusion. These continuous learning processes have resulted in further reductions in actual infections in FY06 to 3 (0.39 infections/1,000 line-days) and an improvement in process reliability to 1 infection in 633 lines through April 30, 2006. The units have not experienced a CLAB since August 14, 2005, despite an 11% increase in admissions, increased acuity, and a near doubling of line use.

Discussion

In the present study, we demonstrated that applying process improvement techniques and system redesign used in industry to the problem of CLABs resulted in rapid, dramatic, and sustainable improvement in clinical outcomes. The findings are in contrast to the results observed when traditional QI efforts were employed. Relying on aggregated, retrospective trend analysis of standardized reports meant that the severity of the problem was not fully appreciated. For example, because extensively used femoral lines were not being counted in the traditional reporting metric, only 19 of the 49 infections met CDC/NNIS reporting criteria. Although the risk of femoral lines remains controversial,[26] it was the most frequent CLAB site in our experience. Furthermore, the reporting of these infections in clinical terms, replete with their dire consequences, motivated workers to engage in process redesign in contrast to the use of complex epidemiological metrics, which were reportable but not actionable. The notion of inevitability is embedded in complex definitions and epidemiological metrics by which the data are generally reported, such as infections/1,000 line-days, which lack clinical context or accountability, and by benchmarking, which implies that there is an acceptable rate.

Moving to a one-by-one identification of variations with real-time problem solving was emotionally difficult. The construction of a clinical vignette about individual cases put nurses and physicians in the position of discussing complications and their potential consequences, with peers, patients, and families. Ongoing education was required for house staff, fellows, and faculty, some of whom challenged openly agreed-upon countermeasures. Such circumstances illustrate the continuous struggle between standardizing practice and the fierce adherence to physician autonomy that constitutes a significant barrier to patient safety efforts in organized medicine.[27] AGH had to contend with issues of status and hierarchy because nurses, by the nature of the direct, continuous care they provide to patients, were most often in a position to identify shortcomings in the methods used by physicians. This meant that the MICU and CCU units had to create a culture and mechanism for drawing attention to problems as they occurred.[28,29]

Despite these concerns, this work provides evidence that CLABs are nearly all preventable when real-time data are used to solve problems as they occur. AGH's experience encourages similar efforts to combat other systemic issues that compromise the delivery of care and demonstrates that the work, properly fostered, can move quickly. Most important, real-time problem solving has transformed the culture from one of blame to one of continuous learning in the pursuit of the elimination of these conditions.

Busy clinicians may see the discipline of real-time problem solving as too time intensive. However, AGH's experience was that solving problems—both in procedure and outcome—as they occurred reduced the need for staff to compensate for ineffective processes (for example, searching for material, information, or help). Having more reliable processes meant that staff members had more time to implement known infection control procedures consistently, and continually improve on them. Patients experienced fewer severe complications that needed time-consuming attention. Taken together, these improvements actually created more time for staff to solve problems and be involved in direct patient care. In addition, the number of admissions to the unit grew steadily without adding new staff or more beds, reflecting greater efficiencies associated with reducing central line infections and their extended length of stay. By focusing on processes, implementation and improvement occurred within 90 days.

LIMITATIONS

There are several limitations in our early work. Specifically, this is a single-center QI initiative employing methods used to eliminate defects in industry to the clinical problem of health care–associated infections. We compared the outcome of this initiative to retrospective results during a comparable period in which traditional

QI approaches based on CDC guidelines were employed. We did not test to see whether the CDC guidelines were being applied with fidelity so we cannot determine conclusively whether our method is better. Our work goes beyond improvement efforts to date that focus principally on issues of proper placement to include a focus on line maintenance as well. The units treated medical intensive care and cardiac patients such that the results may not be applicable to other patient populations (pediatrics, oncology, surgical), although similar improvements have been reported recently from a surgical ICU[30] during a three-year period.

Summary

Real-time problem solving as a method of process improvement was applied to the clinical issue of CLABs in two medical ICUs at AGH. A series of specific, actionable learning activities were created from observations of the care process and real-time analysis of problems. Data were expressed in clinical terms (actual number of patients infected and the risk of infection for central lines) as opposed to using ambiguous epidemiological metrics that tended to conceal the magnitude of the problem and provide little insight into the barriers to improvement. Instead, specific variations in the way care had been delivered prompted staff to make changes in the materials, procedures, and methods of communication used to insert and maintain central venous catheters. These modifications were associated with a 90% reduction in CLABs and a 95% reduction in mortality, sustainable for 34 months. ■

Note: The authors wish to thank Dr. Frank Davidoff for his advice on the manuscript.

References

1. Joint Commission Resources: *Improving Care in the ICU.* Oakbrook Terrace, IL: The Joint Commission, 2004.

2. Mermel L.A.: Prevention of intravascular catheter-related infections. *Ann Intern Med* 132:391–402, Mar. 2000.

3. Vincent J.L.: Nosocomial infections in adult intensive-care units. *Lancet* 361:2068–2077, Jun. 2003.

4. Esen S., Leblebicioglu H.: Prevalence of nosocomial infections at intensive care units in Turkey: A multi-center 1-day point prevalence study. *Scand J Infect Dis* 36(2):144–148, 2004.

5. Verghese S., et al.: Central venous catheter related infections. *J Commun Dis* 31:1–4, Mar. 1999.

6. Maki D.G., Mermel L.A.: Infections due to infusion therapy. In Bennet J.V., Bachman P.S. (eds): *Hospital Infections.* Philadelphia: Lippincott Raven, 1998, pp. 689–724.

7. O'Grady N., et al.: Guidelines for the prevention of intravascular catheter-related infections. *MMWR Recomm Rep* 51(RR-10):1–29, Aug. 9, 2002.

8. Richards M.J., et al.: Nosocomial infections in medical intensive care units in the United States. National Nosocomial Infections Surveillance System. *Crit Care Med* 27:887–892, May 1999.

9. Lieberman M.B., Lau L.J., Williams M.D.: Firm-level productivity and management influence: A comparison of U.S. and Japanese automobile producers. *Management Science* 36:1193–1215, Oct. 1990.

10. Fjimoto T.: *The Evolution of a Manufacturing System at Toyota.* New York: Oxford University Press, 1999.

11. MacDuffie J.P.: The road to root cause: Shop-floor problem-solving at three auto assembly plants. *Management Science* 43:479–502, Apr. 1997.

12. Spear S.J., Bowen H.K.: Decoding the DNA of the Toyota production system. *Harvard Business Review* 77:96–106, Sep.–Oct. 1999.

13. Spear S.J.: The essence of just in time: Embedding diagnostic tests in work-systems to achieve operation excellence. *Production Planning & Control* 13:754–767, Dec. 2002.

14. von Hippel E., Tyre M.: How learning is done: Problem identification in novel process equipment. *Research Policy* 24:1–12, Jan. 1995.

15. Adler P.S., Goldoftas B., Levine D.I.: Flexibility versus efficiency? A case study of model changeovers in the Toyota production system. *Organization Science* 10:43–68, Jan.–Feb. 1999.

16. Clemmer T.P., et al.: Results of a collaborative quality improvement program on outcomes and costs in a tertiary critical care unit. *Crit Care Med* 27:1768–1774, Sep. 1999.

17. Thompson D.N., Wolf G.A., Spear S.J.: Driving improvement in patient care: Lessons from Toyota. *J Nurs Adm* 33:585–595, Nov. 2003.

55

18. Hofer T.P., Hayward R.A.: Are bad outcomes from questionable clinical decisions preventable medical errors? A case of cascade iatrogenesis. *Ann Intern Med* 137:327–333, Sep. 2002.

19. Jaikumar R., Bohn R.E.: Dynamic approach to operations management: An alternative to static optimization. *International Journal of Production Economics* 27:265–282, Oct. 1992.

20. Adler P.S., Cole R.E.: Designed for learning: A tale of two auto plants. *Sloan Manage Rev* 34:85–94, Spring 1993.

21. Institute for Healthcare Improvement: *Putting Safety on the Central Line.* http://www.ihi.org/IHI/Topics/CriticalCare/IntensiveCare/ImprovementStories/PuttingSafet yontheCentralLine.htm (accessed Jan. 25, 2007).

22. Institute for Healthcare Improvement: *Frequently Asked Questions about the 5 Million Lives Campaign.* http://www.ihi.org/IHI/Programs/Campaign/Campaign.htm?TabId=6 (accessed Jan. 25, 2007).

23. Sirio C.A., et al.: Pittsburgh Regional Healthcare Initiative: A systems approach for achieving perfect patient care. *Health Aff (Millwood)* 22:157–165, Sep.–Oct. 2003.

24. Reduction in central line–associated bloodsteam infections among patients in intensive care units–Pennsylvania. April 2001–March 2005. *MMWR Morb Mortal Wkly Rep* 54:1013–1016, Oct. 14, 2005.

25. Grunden, N.: Industrial techniques help reduce hospital-acquired infection. Biomed *Instrum Technol* 39:307–311, Sep.–Oct. 2005.

26. Deshpande K.S., et al.: The incidence of infectious complications of central venous catheters at the subclavian, internal jugular, and femoral sites in an intensive care unit population. *Crit Care Med* 33:13–20, Jan. 2005.

27. Reinertsen J.: Zen and the art of physician autonomy maintenance. *Ann Intern Med* 140:585, Apr. 2004.

28. Edmondson A.C.: Learning from mistakes is easier said than done: Group and organizational influences on the detection and correction of human error. *J Applied Beh Sci* 40(1):66–90, 2004.

29. Tucker A.L., Edmondson A.E., Spear S.J.: When problem solving prevents organizational learning. *Journal of Organizational Change Management* 15:122–137, Apr. 2002.

30. Berenholtz S.M., et al.: Eliminating catheter-related bloodstream infections in the intensive care unit. *Crit Care Med* 32:2014–2020, Oct. 2004.

This chapter first appeared in the September 2006 (Volume 32, Number 9, pages 479–487) issue of *The Joint Commission Journal on Quality and Patient Safety.*

Evidence-Based Practice to Reduce Central Line Infections

Marta L. Render, M.D.

Suzanne Brungs, R.N.

Uma Kotagal, M.D.

Mary Nicholson, R.N.

Patricia Burns, R.N.

Deborah Ellis, R.N.

Marla Clifton, R.N.

Rosie Fardo, R.N.

Mark Scott, M.D.

Larry Hirschhorn, Ph.D.

The greater metropolitan area of Cincinnati includes three states (Indiana, Kentucky, and Ohio) and 14 counties with slightly more than two million people (http://www.the-collaborative.org/files/ demooverview.pdf.) The Greater Cincinnati Health Council (GCHC) initially coordinated hospital concerns about public health issues, such as clean water. GCHC now provides neutral ground for its 35 hospital members (representing about 230,000 discharges in 2003) to address changes in today's health care environment. Through the GCHC, hospitals, employers, insurers, and patients collaborate to improve community health, consolidate data services, promote health education, and reduce costs through group purchasing among other services. For example, members of the council's patient safety and pharmacy work groups standardized implementation of surgical site marking and abbreviation use in med-

About the Authors

Marta L. Render, M.D., is Chief, VA Inpatient Evaluation Center (IPEC), Veterans Affairs Medical Center, Cincinnati, and Project Leader for the Greater Cincinnati Health Council Collaborative for Patient Safety.

Suzanne Brungs, R.N., is Project Coordinator, IPEC, Veterans Affairs Medical Center, Cincinnati.

Uma Kotagal, M.D., is Vice President for Quality and Transformation, Cincinnati Children's Hospital Medical Center, Cincinnati.

Mary Nicholson, R.N., is an Infection Control Practitioner, Christ Hospital, Cincinnati.

Patricia Burns, R.N., is an Infection Control Practitioner, St. Elizabeth Medical Center, Edgewood, Kentucky.

Deborah Ellis, R.N., is an Infection Control Practitioner, St. Elizabeth Medical Center, Edgewood, Kentucky.

Marla Clifton, R.N., is an Infection Control Practitioner, Jewish Hospital, Cincinnati.

Rosie Fardo, R.N., is the Infection Control Specialist and Safety Officer, Mercy Mount Airy Hospital, Cincinnati.

Mark Scott, M.D., is Director of the Medical Intensive Care Unit, Christ Hospital, Cincinnati.

Larry Hirschhorn, Ph.D., is a Principal, Center for Applied Research, Philadelphia.

Please address reprint requests to Marta L. Render, marta.render@med.va.gov.

ical orders and records. In 2003, the GCHC president solicited commitment by leaders of nine health care systems to jointly fund a project to reduce hospital-acquired infections, which was developed by a patient safety researcher [M.L.R.] at Veterans Affairs Medical Center, Cincinnati. The objective of the project was to implement evidence-based patient safety practices that reduce surgical site infections (SIP)—surgical antibiotic prophylaxis timing, temperature, glycemic control—and catheter-related blood stream infections (CR-BSIs)—chorhexidine and maximal sterile barriers—at the nine health care systems' 10 hospitals during a two-year period and train hospital staff in methods to successfully create and sustain change. Experts in organizational change [U.K., L.H.] facilitated practice change strategies. The project targeted reduction of hospital-acquired infections for the following reasons:

1. Recommendations to reduce hospital-acquired infections are well studied and largely accepted.
2. Substantial variability exists in the adoption of most of these practices.
3. Hospitals have accepted and defined roles and responsibility to minimize hospital-acquired infections.
4. The process change might improve both patient and economic outcomes for the hospitals. A hospital-acquired infection is one that occurs > 48 hours after admission to the hospital and < 72 hours following discharge. Hospital-acquired infections occur in 7%–10% of hospitalized patients, account for 80,000 deaths a year in the United States, and lead to approximately $3.5 billion in direct costs per year.[1-8] In addition, only a small percentage (9%) of preventable hospital-acquired infections are actually prevented.[1] This article describes the part of the project that won the Codman Award: implementation of evidence-based practices that rapidly reduced CR-BSIs. A CR-BSI is defined as a positive blood culture with clinical or microbiologic evidence that strongly implicates the catheter as the source of infection.[8] It is distinguished from local infection (evidence of purulence at the site of insertion) and catheter colonization (growth of greater than 15 colony forming units of an organism from the tip or subcutaneous portion of the catheter using the semiquantitative roll-plate culture technique).[9] CR-BSI affects more than 200,000 patients a year in the United States[10,11] increasing mortality risk from 4% to 35%[12-14] and costing an estimated $6,000–$40,000 per episode.[14,15] A recent quantitative review found that 25% of patients develop catheter colonization, and 5% develop CR-BSI, with an average catheter placement of eight days.[14] The Centers

for Disease Control and Prevention (CDC) reports CR-BSI rates that range from 2.8 to 12.8 infections per 1,000 catheter days for all types of intensive care units (ICUs).[16] Strict adherence to proper hand washing,[17,18] maximum barrier precautions (sterile gown and gloves, cap, mask, bed-size sterile drape), and use of chlorhexidine gluconate antiseptic instead of betadine during placement reduces CR-BSI. A randomized controlled trial of 343 patients, comparing maximum sterile barrier (MSB) (sterile gloves, long-sleeved sterile gown, a full bed-size drape, and nonsterile mask and cap) to usual practice (use of sterile gloves and sterile small drape) found significantly different rates of CR-BSI (0.08/1,000 line-days versus 0.5/1,000 line-days, $p = .02$).[19] Despite the additional costs of a large drape and chlorhexidine, use of MSB has been estimated to be cost-saving in simplified "back-of-the-envelope" cost studies.[20]

Methods

SETTING
The nine health care systems and 10 hospitals represented federal, university, tertiary care referral, suburban, and rural hospitals and a children's hospital (*see* Table 4-1). The project was reviewed by each hospital's Institutional Review Board.

TEAMS
At project initiation, each hospital's CEO and other hospital leaders identified the project leader and team members. The hospital infection control professional often led the team, which consisted of the nurse manager of the intervention unit, two or more staff nurses, a physician champion, and the supply manager. Although they were all invited to the kickoff by the project leader, the number of team members participating varied from only the team leader (the infection control practitioner) to eight or more team members. The leadership role of the infection control practitioners, which was assigned by the CEOs, proved important because they already knew and believed the literature, had previously collaborated outside the confines of their own hospital, understood the data collection issues, and had some flexibility in their schedules.

INTERVENTION
Health care systems were randomized to begin their intervention either in the operating room or in the intensive care unit (medical ICU if > 1 ICU was present).

TABLE 4-1. Hospital Characteristics

Characteristic	Intervention	Control
Number of hospitals	4	5
Annual discharges (acute care)	83,636	100,864
Hospital type		
University	—	1
Urban referral	2	1
Federal	—	1
Suburban	2	2
Affiliation with national health care organization	1	1
Intensive care units (total *N*)	8	13
Intensive care unit beds	104	169
Central line days/year	7,714	3,978

Source: Authors.

Kickoff. At a joint 1.5-day session, national experts presented the evidence for the practices, while experts in organizational change presented the methods for change and mentored the teams' implementation planning. The teams were to come up with the following:
- A SMART aim (one that was specific, measurable, actionable, reliable, and time driven)
- A 90-day goal, with communication strategy, measurement, and tests of change
- A 3-day itemized action plan that addressed recruitment of additional team members, the first test of change, and roles

Work-Learning-Reporting Cycles. Project leaders organized the work-learning-reporting cycles at each site, which included at minimum one test of change each month (initially very small). Together, they met monthly with project leadership and reported their experience using a standardized format (six presentation slides in small groups [< 10 people]) to share effective strategies, solve similar sorts of problems together, reinforce the change theory and methodology, and develop consistent data collection strategies and definitions.

PROJECT COMMUNICATION

Each project leader reported processes and outcomes to the unit staff, usually posting the monthly project presentation slides on a bulletin board throughout the unit. Results were also reported through the preexisting hospital committee structure (for example, surgical service committee, infection control, critical care committee) in each organization and to the hospital as a whole through its newsletter. At the community level, project leadership reported outcomes of the project to the GCHC infection control and patient safety committees. Twice a year, project leadership informed the hospital CEOs of the results of the project, which compared local process adherence and outcomes to the mean of the group.

MEASUREMENT

Central lines were defined as any intravenous catheter whose distal end was in a central vein. Beginning in January 2004 and to continue through December 2006, nurses in the ICUs used a checklist (*see* Appendix 1) that offered binary choices (yes/no) for hand washing, chlorhexidine use, bed-size sterile drape, and use by the operator of cap/mask/sterile gown/sterile gloves during insertion, as well as date and site of catheter. After the date of removal was entered, the checklists were then forwarded to the project leader and the data were collated and entered into a secure deidentified Web-based database. To ascertain capture of all central lines, nurse managers each month sampled the lines in place in the ICU against the forms.

Outcomes Measures. At the project's inception, all hospitals were already collecting CR-BSI data using the CDC definitions. After ensuring standardization of the definitions across the hospitals, infection control professionals at both the CR-BSI intervention hospitals and the SIP hospitals reported CR-BSIs and line-days stratified by ICU (CR-BSI; x per 1,000 line-days) to the project.

Barrier and Facilitator Identification. After six months, the project leader [M.R.] and project coordinator [S.B.] reviewed their detailed notes from the monthly reporting meetings to independently identify themes contributing to or delaying project success. The list of barriers and facilitators was then validated by the project leaders.

ANALYSIS

Outcome Analysis. We compared CR-BSI rates from 2004 with CR-BSI rates from 2003 at intervention and control ICUs. As a sensitivity analysis, we compared pre– and post–line-days using a *t*-test because an increase in the denominator (reflecting more accurate collection of line-days) alone would decrease the infection rate, which is reported as a fraction.

Process Analysis. We tracked adherence to individual practices over time.

Results

The four hospitals that started the ICU project in 2004 set a goal to reduce their CR-BSI rates by 50%.

DEMOGRAPHICS

During the first year of the project, a total of 742 lines were placed in the 686 patients at the four hospitals for 10,472 line-days. The lines stayed in for a mean of 7.0 ± 6.2 days. Of these lines, 27% were urgent, 60% were multiple lumen catheters, and 25% were placed in the femoral vein.

PROCESS CHANGES

Hospitals used a checklist and forcing functions to standardize insertion of central lines. The checklist was completed by nursing as the physician prepares for the procedure, acting as both a teaching and a measurement tool. Within the first week, project leaders determined that all commercially available central line trays included a small drape and both chlorhexidine and betadine, allowing practitioners to easily avoid practice change. Collaborating with two manufacturers, the team leaders modified the prepackaged insertion trays (removing the betadine and small drape) and developed an "accessory pack" that bundled the large drape, the sterile gown, and cap and mask. The tray, accessory pack, and sterile gloves were all accessed with the checklist on a central line cart—making it easy to do it right. In most units, betadine was removed. Finally, to promote sustained practice change, hospital committees at the senior leadership level (clinical executive board) also approved written policies that matched the best practices to codify the practice change.

OUTCOMES

Process Adherence. Initially, no site used a sterile drape that covered the entire bed. Chlorhexidine, despite its availability in the central line tray, was used less than 50% of the time. Gloves were the only element of the bundle used every time by every practitioner. Process adherence increased from 0 (for bed-size sterile drapes) to 85%–95% (*see* Figure 4-1).

CR-BSIs. As process adherence increased, the CR-BSI rates in the medical ICUs of all four hospitals fell more than 50% from 1.7/1,000 line-days to 0.4 per 1,000 line- days ($p < .05$, *see* Figure 4-2, page 64). In fact, infection rates were 0 in three of the four hospitals for four quarters.

FIGURE 4-1. Process Adherence Increased for both Chlorhexidine and Bed-Size Sterile Drapes

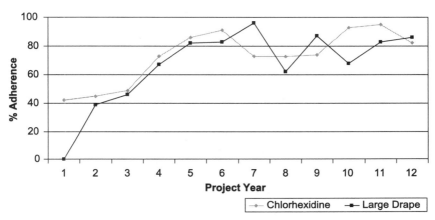

Adherence to Process Changes—Chlorhexidine and Large Drape
Source: Authors.

Barriers/Facilitators. Hospital and project leadership, previous experience in project implementation, measurement, change methodology, communication strategies (*see,* for example, Figure 4-3), and approaches that increased pull or motivation of the clinical staff, as well as project locus external to the hospital and extending across multiple local hospitals were all important facilitators and barriers to implementation of the CR-BSI project; they are detailed in Table 4-2. The following four elements deserve comment:

1. The important role played by hospital leadership cannot be overestimated; the success and the time line to success at these hospitals was directly related to the ways that leadership visibly communicated commitment to this project.
2. Feedback of early measurement is critical, even before the project begins.
3. The rapid action cycle is not well understood across acute care inpatient units and is contrary to the usual medical epidemiologic model (measure and plan everything forever first). Conversion to this change method speeds up conversion to new practices.
4. The external locus of the project from each hospital's management prevented delay and decay in the project despite leadership changes at the middle and senior level.

FIGURE 4-2. Catheter-Related Blood Stream Infection (CR-BSI) Rates

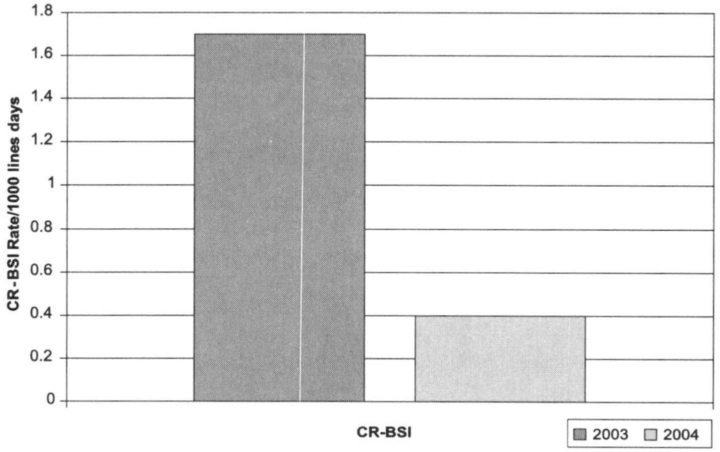

Catheter-related blood stream infection rates were reduced at intensive care units that implemented the bundle of practices.
Source: Authors.

Discussion

The results of this project surprised participants. First, the reduction of central line infection rates initially to zero and then persistently below 1/1,000 line-days was unexpected, suggesting that the low end of the present benchmark is overestimated. Next, the utility of the rapid action cycle, with the need to get each element of the process right in small tests of change before broad dissemination, was apparent to all. Finally, the ease and benefit of local collaboration using home-grown change leaders who were grounded in the latest art of change seems noteworthy.

Until this initiative, all participants had active infection control programs and assumed that their CR-BSI rates were unavoidable, particularly because our aggregated rates were below the reported 25th percentile (range, 1.9 to 3.7 CR-BSI/1,000 line-days) from the 1992–2004 published rates in medical or medical surgical ICUs in hospitals participating in the National Nosocomial Infection Surveillance Database.[21] Most project leaders voiced skepticism regarding their ability to drive the CR-BSI rates down, even after identification of significant variation in the use of sterile gown/mask/cap, large drapes, and chlorhexidine during central catheter insertion.[22]

TABLE 4-2. Barriers and Facilitators*

Project	Facilitators	Barriers
Hospital leadership	CEO directive to team and to hospital staff	Prioritization of practice change, "get to it when we can, first we need to use the 250 forms we made up in 1997 . . ."
	Project external to the organization proved powerful for continuity	Changes in middle or senior management
Experience	Building on prior pilot	"Myth of perfection"
Measurement	Measurement of process and outcomes with feedback	Comparison with benchmark creates a floor ("acceptable or good infection rate")
Change method	The "right" team	
	Applying rapid cycle change with campaign strategy	Epidemiologic model ("I need more data, let's collect data for another month")
Communication	Advertising change and its success in hospital news "2 minutes to save a life"	
	Comparison of local hospital with aggregate performance	
	Local celebration of success	
Project leadership	Infection control professional with experience in implementation, M.D. champion, local leadership in loop	Stovepiped responsibility and expertise; example: infection control professional as a consultant/epidemiologist, not a change agent.
		Distributed authority and conflicting goals stymied process. Example: Supply's performance goal is cost containment.

continued on page 66

65

TABLE 4-2. Barriers and Facilitators*, *continued*

Project	Facilitators	Barriers
Motivation Multiple sites	Match personal/organizational agendas to project (nursing ladder, publication/presentation)	
	Learning across the hospitals; peer problem solving reduces frustration/fatigue	Isolation, conflicting goals (multiple quality projects in all hospitals)
	Reduction in rework (example: advertising, slogans, strategy to recruit M.D. champion)	Reward based on individual performance
	Celebrating success as a unit	
	Deadlines for reporting (monthly storyboard meetings)	

* CEO, chief executive officer; M.D., physician.

Source: Authors

The simultaneous reduction of CR-BSI rates to 0 across multiple hospitals in a single metropolitan area with implementation of evidence-based processes had not been reported, although a recent investigation in a single institution described reduction of CR-BSI rates to 0 with multifaceted interventions.[23]

Use of a rapid action cycle, with small tests of change, and huddles to evaluate, learn, and adapt the process until "right" was new to many in these hospitals. The hospitals were expected to implement in a very small way some process change the very next week, adopting a slogan of "what can you do by Tuesday." Testing parts of the intervention first with a single helpful practitioner allows missteps to be corrected without sabotaging the effort. The selection of only a small group of practitioners to collaborate initially in the change process also created cachet for the project. As the project progressed, reports of monthly process adherence alongside falling infection rates minimized resistance. The purchase of the modified central line trays and accessory packs reduced the effort necessary for process adherence, improving practice reliability. Similar success has been described with use of corporate performance improvement models.[24]

FIGURE 4-3. Poster for Process Changes to Reduce Central Line Infections

Reduce central line infections

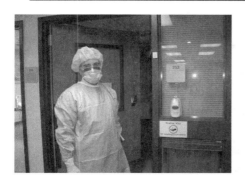

Alcohol Hand Gel. . 10 seconds

Maximum Sterile
Barriers . . . . .50 seconds

Chloraprep. .Apply. .30 seconds
Dry. . . . 30 seconds
_____

2 minutes

Marketing the process changes to clinical staff created pull; a poster created at one of the hospitals was used by a total of 5 of the 10 hospitals is shown.
Source: Authors.

Hospitals in most communities privately manage their patient safety problems, rarely sharing their experience with other hospitals. This narrow approach to patient safety prevents spread of lessons from one hospital to another. Such sharing might avoid the requirement of patient injury as the impetus for practice change.[25] Implementation of evidence-based patient safety practices through a community collaborative appeared to reduce pushback from practitioners, rework, and the cost of the initiatives through sharing of products and processes to promote learning. Hospitals adopted and adapted measurement tools, marketing and communication strategies (*see* Figure 4-3), training modules, and shared methods to promote the project, speaking to the benefit of this model. The collaborative used group advocacy to develop the modified central line insertion tray with manufacturers, and provided support external to the hospital when the project was struggling either as a result of change in management or multiple other competing goals. Part of the success of this strategy might lie in the comparative feedback regarding CR-BSI rates as opposed to using information about internal rates alone as had been described by others.[26] ■

Note: A portion of the data reported in this article was reported at the American Thoracic Society Meeting, San Diego, May 23–24, 2005.

APPENDIX 4-1. Intensive Care Unit (ICU) Line Insertion Check Sheet

FILL OUT FOR ALL LINE INSERTIONS

Insertion Date: _____ Time: _____
Type of line: _____ Site: _____
Guide wire change _____ Yes _____ No
Non-urgent _____ Urgent/emergency _____

ADDRESSOGRAPH

OBSERVATIONS	R-1	R-2	R-3	ATTENDING	PICC RN
WASH/DISINFECT HANDS	YES NO	YES NO	YES NO	YES NO	YES NO
HEAD COVER	YES NO	YES NO	YES NO	YES NO	YES NO
MASK	YES NO	YES NO	YES NO	YES NO	YES NO
CHLORAPREP SWAB	YES NO	YES NO	YES NO	YES NO	YES NO
STERILE SURGEON GOWN	YES NO	YES NO	YES NO	YES NO	YES NO
STERILE GLOVES	YES NO	YES NO	YES NO	YES NO	YES NO
FULL BODY DRAPE	YES NO	YES NO	YES NO	YES NO	YES NO
SONA SITE/SITE RITE	YES NO	YES NO	YES NO	YES NO	YES NO
PROBE COVER	YES NO	YES NO	YES NO	YES NO	YES NO

FAX COPY TO   ; ORIGINAL – PLACE IN   'S MAILBOX
THANK YOU!

Hospital Admission date   _____   ICU admission date: _____
Hospital Discharge date   _____   ICU discharge date: _____

Line removal date _____ Infection _____ No _____ Yes

Type: _____ *CR-BSI*[*] _____ *Lab confirmed bacteremia* _____ *exit site infection* _____ *colonized cath tip*

[*] CR-BSI, catheter-related bloodstream infection.
Source: Authors.

References

1. Haley R.W., et al.: The efficacy of infection surveillance and control programs in preventing nosocomial infections in US hospitals. *Am J Epidemiol* 121:182–205, Feb. 1985.

2. Jarvis W.R.: Selected aspects of the socioeconomic impact of nosocomial infections: Morbidity, mortality, cost, and prevention. *Infect Control Hosp Epidemiol* 17:552–557, Aug. 1996.

3. Richards M.J., et al.: Nosocomial infections in medical intensive care units in the United States. National Nosocomial Infections Surveillance System. *Crit Care Med* 27:887–892, May 1999.

4. National Nosocomial Infections Surveillance (NNIS) report, data summary from October 1986–April 1997, issued May 1997. A report from the NNIS System. *Am J Infect Control* 25:477–487, Dec. 1997.

5. National Nosocomial Infections Surveillance (NNIS) report, data summary from October 1986–April 1996, issued May 1996: A report from the National Nosocomial Infections Surveillance (NNIS) System. *Am J Infect Control* 24:380–388, Oct. 1996.

6. Martone W.J., et al.: National Nosocomial Infections Surveillance (NNIS) semiannual report, May 1995: A report from the National Nosocomial Infections Surveillance (NNIS) System. *Am J Infect Control* 23:377–385, Dec. 1995.

7. Horan T.C., et al.: Nosocomial infections in surgical patients in the United States, January 1986–June 1992. National Nosocomial Infections Surveillance (NNIS) System. *Infect Control Hosp Epidemiol* 14:73–80, Feb. 1993.

8. Raad I.I., Bodey G.P.: Infectious complications of indwelling vascular catheters. *Clin Infect Dis* 15:197–208, Aug. 1992.

9. Maki D.G., Weise C.E., Sarafin H.W.: A semiquantitative culture method for identifying intravenous-catheter-related infection. *N Engl J Med* 296:1305–1309, Jun. 9, 1977.

10. Saint S., Veentra D.L., Lipsky B.A.: The clinical and economic consequences of nosocomial central venous catheter-related infection: Are antimicrobial catheters useful? *Infect Control Hosp Epidemiol* 21:375–380, Jun. 2000.

11. Maki D.G.: Infections caused by intravascular devices used for infusion therapy. In Bistro A.I., Waldvogel F.A. (eds.): *Infections Associated with Indwelling Medical Devices.* Washington, DC, ASM Press, 1994, pp. 155–205.

12. Soufir L., et al.: Attributable morbidity and mortality of catheter-related septicemia in critically ill patients: A matched, risk-adjusted, cohort study. *Infect Control Hosp Epidemiol* 20:396–401, Jun. 1999.

13. Pittet D., Tarara D., Wenzel R.P.: Nosocomial bloodstream infection in critically ill patients: Excess length of stay, extra costs, and attributable mortality. *JAMA* 271:1598–1601, May 25, 1994.

14. Saint S.: Clinical and economic consequences of nosocomial catheter-related bacteriuria. *Am J Infect Control* 28:68–75, Feb. 2000.

15. Pittet D., Wenzel R.P.: Nosocomial bloodstream infections. Secular trends in rates, mortality, and contribution to total hospital deaths. *Arch Intern Med* 155:1177–1184, Jun. 1995.

16. National Nosocomial Infections Surveillance (NNIS) System report, data summary from October 1986–April 1998, issued June 1998. *Am J Infect Control* 26:522–533, Oct. 1998.

17. Nystrom B.: Impact of handwashing on mortality in intensive care: Examination of the evidence. *Infect Control Hosp Epidemiol* 15:435–436, Jul. 1994.

18. Doebbeling B.N., et al.: Comparative efficacy of alternative handwashing agents in reducing nosocomial infections in intensive care units. *N Engl J Med* 327:88–93, Jul. 9, 1992.

19. Raad I.I., et al.: Prevention of central venous catheter-related infections by using maximal sterile barrier precautions during insertion. *Infect Control Hosp Epidemiol* 15(4 pt. 1):231–238, Apr. 1994.

20. Sherertz R.J., et al.: Education of physicians-in-training can decrease the risk for vascular catheter infection. *Ann Intern Med* 132:641–648, Apr. 2000.

21. National Nosocomial Infections Surveillance (NNIS) System Report, data summary from January 1992 through June 2004, issued October 2004. *Am J Infect Control* 32:470–485, Dec. 2004.

22. Braun B.I., et al: Preventing central venous catheter-associated primary bloodstream infections: Characteristics of practices among hospitals participating in the Evaluation of Processes and Indicators in Infection Control (EPIC) study. *Infect Control Hosp Epidemiol* 24:926–935, Dec. 2003.

23. Berenholtz S.M., et al.: Eliminating catheter-related bloodstream infections in the intensive care unit. *Crit Care Med* 32:2014–2020, Oct. 2004.

24. Frankel H.L., et al.: Use of corporate Six Sigma performance-improvement strategies to reduce incidence of catheter-related bloodstream infections in a surgical ICU. *J Am Coll Surg* 201:349–358, Sep. 2005.

25. Institute of Medicine: *To Err Is Human: Building a Safer Health System.* Washington, DC: National Academy Press, 1999.

26. McKinley L.L., et al.: Effect of comparative data feedback on intensive care unit infection rates in a Veterans Administration Hospital Network System. *Am J Infect Control* 31:397–404, Nov. 2003.

This chapter first appeared in the May 2006 (Volume 32, Number 5, pages 253–260) issue of *The Joint Commission Journal on Quality and Patient Safety.*

Monitoring Patient Safety in Health Care: Building the Case for Surrogate Measures

Robert P. Gaynes, M.D.
Richard Platt, M.D.

W e live in the age of measurement in health care that drives both care and reimbursement. Remarkably, objective measurements of patient safety remain difficult to develop. Lee and colleagues recently described a pressing need for the medical community to engage with payers, purchasers, and patients in developing meaningful and broadly applicable measures of the quality of health care.[1] Such measures are notably lacking for many adverse health events, which have been the target of great interest and activity, especially since the publication of the Institute of Medicine's report *To Err Is Human*.[2,3]

About the Authors

Robert P. Gaynes, M.D., is Assistant to the Director, Division of Healthcare Quality Promotion, Centers for Disease Control and Prevention, Atlanta, and Associate Professor, Emory University School of Medicine, Atlanta.

Richard Platt, M.D., is Professor and Chair, Department of Ambulatory Care and Prevention, Harvard Medical School and Harvard Pilgrim Health Care, and Professor of Medicine and Hospital Epidemiologist, Brigham and Women's Hospital and Harvard Medical School, Boston.

Please address correspondence to Robert P. Gaynes, M.D., rpg1@cdc.gov.

We describe a new approach to monitoring adverse events in health care with a focus on hospital-associated infections because they are major health care safety problems. More than one million hospital-acquired infections occur each year in the United States, of which thousands are fatal.[4] In addition, infection control programs that are designed to identify and prevent these infections are among the oldest, best-developed, and most frequently cited quality measurement activities.[5] We concentrate on infections that occur in nonoutbreak situations because they account for at least 90% of hospital-acquired infections.[6] They are also the infections that are most relevant for assessing performance over time or across facilities. Despite all the monitoring of such infections, there are no known objective measures associated with preventable outcomes that most health care facilities can use as benchmarks.

Influences on Surveillance

There have been three major influences on surveillance of hospital-associated (previously called hospital-acquired or nosocomial) infections in the United States. The landmark Study on the Efficacy of Nosocomial Infection Control [SENIC] Project) concluded that effective infection control programs must include active surveillance (characterized by systematic assessment that uses standard definitions rather than reliance on spontaneous reporting by clinicians) coupled with prevention/control activities, an adequate number of trained infection control staff, and a system for dissemination of surveillance data, that is, reporting surgical site infection (SSI) rates to surgeons.[7] The findings of the SENIC Project provided the scientific basis for the assertion that surveillance tied to effort in prevention/control is an essential element of a quality improvement (QI) program. The relevance remains. Indeed, no other component of quality assurance has, as its basis, a scientific study from a probability sample of 338 hospitals in the United States.

The second influence on current surveillance programs came in 1976, when The Joint Commission issued a recommendation, largely on the basis of the SENIC Project's findings, that hospitals have one infection control practitioner per 250 beds. Although that ratio's relevance is decidedly uncertain today, the staffing increases that occurred in response to that recommendation placed infection control programs in the United States in an enviable position—infection surveillance/control programs hired trained personnel to perform active surveillance. Active surveillance outperforms spontaneous reporting of infections or other events,[8] not only because spontaneous reporting typically identifies a minority of events of interest but also because the undocumented reporting biases can distort observed trends in the incidence of disease, prevent accurate assessment of benefits or impact of control programs, or prevent timely identification of disease outbreaks.[8] In spite of these problems, considerable energy is currently devoted to enhancing the amount of spontaneous reporting of adverse events.[9] Yet we believe the emphasis should be placed on the much more important need to develop rate-based, uniform, active surveillance methods that would yield comparable results in different settings.

Unfortunately, active surveillance for hospital-associated infections has been a time-consuming process, requiring nearly half of infection control practitioners' time.[10,11] Although hospitals allocate substantial resources to measurement of hospital-associated infections, most health care organizations cannot effectively monitor all of the important infections or other aspects of the care they provide.[12] In addition, surveillance absorbs time and resources that could be used for other essential components of an effective infection control program, such as prevention and QI activities.

The third major influence on surveillance in the United States was the Centers for Disease Control and Prevention (CDC)'s National Nosocomial Infections Surveillance (NNIS) system. The NNIS system began in 1970, when selected hospitals began voluntarily and confidentially reporting their hospital-associated infection surveillance data for aggregation into a national database.[13] Through the NNIS system, infections are monitored using standardized methodology and categorized into major and specific infection sites, using CDC definitions that include laboratory and clinical criteria.[14] To meet CDC definitions for infection, infection control practitioners perform a two-step process: (1) screening for possible cases of infection, often by a review of microbiology records, and (2) confirmation, typically by a complete patient record review. This process is required to confirm a clinical infection and is required for many other adverse health events; for example, a significant bleeding event after warfarin dosing. The NNIS approach to surveillance achieved some success. The CDC reported substantial reductions in hospital-associated infection rates from intensive care units among hospitals that participated in the NNIS system, suggesting the value of the NNIS system in preventing hospital-associated infections.[15]

Some experts have recommended this model for assessing other adverse events associated with hospital care.[16] Indeed, as of this writing the states of Florida, Illinois, Missouri, Nevada, Pennsylvania, New York, and Virginia are mandating hospitals to publicly report their infection rates using NNIS or related methods (*see*, for example, Illinois Public Act 93-0563, and Missouri HCS/SS/SCS/SB 1279-Missouri Nosocomial Infection Control Act of 2004).

Despite the NNIS model's value, important drawbacks limit its use. First, screening for adverse events is challenging. For example, because of decreasing postoperative stays, a majority of SSIs are missed if a formal postdischarge surveillance system is not in place.[17] However, there is no agreed-on method for SSI detection in the outpatient area.[18–31] Second, many NNIS definitions can be satisfied by a physician's diagnosis,[13] despite the fact that clinicians vary both in the criteria they use to diagnose a hospital-associated infection and in the completeness of their documentation of these events. Thus, the NNIS system's attempt to capture clinicians' thinking has resulted in "standard" definitions with variable and nonreproducible criteria. Finally, inadequate methods for risk adjustment limit the value of data using the NNIS model for benchmarking.[32] The NNIS system and others like it are caught between the ongoing demand for better, more detailed measures and the lack of resources to provide them.

Developing Objective and Universal Measures

We need a new approach because an essential tenet of the current goal of surveillance—focusing only on rigorously confirmed adverse events—is neither necessary nor achievable across the entire health care system. Efforts should be directed instead to creating acceptably accurate objective measures of quality of care and of outcomes that can be used by all health care facilities.

Two major principles should guide the development of the new measures. First, the measures should evaluate the same event, no matter where the care is delivered or who collects the information. Second, every hospital, health care provider, or payer should be able to implement the measures relevant to the care provided or compensated. To achieve the first principle, it would be necessary to use more objective measures—ones that do not force the monitor to get inside the head of the clinician. To achieve the second, we should make greater use of the vast amount of information that is already being routinely created during the delivery of health care, and that therefore requires little, if any, additional resources of clinicians, infection control practitioners, or other QI personnel.

Adopting objective measures would be easier if we are open to two kinds of alternatives—(1) process measures that correlate with infections or other adverse outcomes of health care and (2) surrogate measures of important outcomes.

Process Measures

Process measures, as their name implies, assess the delivery of care rather than the outcomes. They can be useful when their link to beneficial or adverse outcomes is well established. Appropriate delivery of perioperative antibiotic prophylaxis, a measure of surgical quality now being implemented by The Joint Commission, is an example of a process measure that emerged from decades of research.[33] Limiting the frequency and duration of use of indwelling urinary catheters is another example of a process measure that is correlated with fewer urinary tract infections. Although the details of the specific yardstick may be debated, process measures must be coupled to an important outcome and be directly amenable to improvement. In addition, because health care–associated infections and adverse health outcomes occur much less commonly than problems in process, measuring the process of care provides many more opportunities to identify and remedy suboptimal performance before patients suffer the consequences.

Surrogate Measures

Surrogate measures of interest for infection surveillance are ones that measure objective, readily ascertained events that are sufficiently correlated with infections to provide useful information about organizations' actual infection rates. Such measures may hold even greater value than process measures for benchmarking organizations.

Like process measures, surrogate measures must also be connected to an essential and preventable outcome of interest. Surrogate measures have become standards in clinical medicine—for example, glycosolated hemoglobin (A1C). Clinicians use hemoglobin A1C as a surrogate to monitor control of diabetes mellitus on the basis of decades of research that show its relevance to improved outcomes.[34] We have only started to identify such surrogates for organizational performance in hospital epidemiology, but there are some. For example, the SSI rate following coronary artery bypass, cesarean section, and breast surgery appears to correlate closely enough with the proportion of patients who receive extended courses of inpatient antibiotics to be a useful indicator of a hospital's outcomes for those procedures.[35-37] Monitoring the proportion of patients who exceed a procedure-specific number of days of antibiotic exposure would allow us to identify hospitals or patient groups that merit closer attention to determine whether their infection rates or their antibiotic usage patterns are high. Such surrogates should not be equated with the actual outcomes we wish to prevent. Our goal would not necessarily be to reduce the number of patients who receive long courses of postoperative antibiotics, for example, stimulating clinicians to shorten the antibiotic courses they prescribe in management of infections. Surrogate measures are analogous to the screening step that is part of current surveillance activities. The major difference we propose, compared to current surveillance practice, is that we would require surrogate measures to contain sufficient information by themselves so that we would not need to confirm every event that they detect. For example, investigators at one medical center found that a computer algorithm to detect bloodstream infections outperformed manual chart review.[38]

Simplifying the approach to monitoring bloodstream infection surveillance using this computer algorithm or other approaches[39] would allow infection control practitioners more time to focus on other surveillance or prevention activities. Objective surrogate measures would reduce interobserver variation and the need for specialized training and could be used across a wide range of health care organizations, making some of them attractive candidates for interhospital comparison and possibly more attractive than outcome measures currently recommended by the Healthcare Infection Control Practices Advisory Committee (HICPAC),[40] such as central line–associated, laboratory-confirmed bloodstream infections or SSIs, each of which has limitations.[40]

Research is essential to develop new surrogate measures of health care–associated infections and to test their performance characteristics, that is, to understand whether they identify a sufficient fraction of outcomes of interest (sensitivity) with an acceptably low number of false positives (specificity or predictive value). The new surrogate measures that would be most useful are those that can be constructed from data that are available in automated form as part of routine health care delivery. Such surrogate measures would facilitate the development of standard reporting systems that health care providers or payers can implement with relatively little cost.

Automated health care data have been used to detect hospital-associated infections[38,41] and other detrimental health outcomes such as adverse drug events and patient falls.[42] Although complete computerized patient records are currently available in only a minority of health care organizations, computerized diagnosis, procedure, and pharmacy billing data are very widely available. Appropriate caution has already been sounded regarding the use of such administrative data to detect adverse health events,[43] but we believe that prudent use of selected data can provide consistent and substantially better information about hospital-associated infections and possibly other safety problems than is currently available.

The information that payers hold may become crucial because hospitals and ambulatory care facilities simply do not have much of the required information about postdischarge care. Some progress has been made in developing surrogate measures of hospital-associated infections by using payers' data. For SSIs, promising surrogate measures that are more efficient than traditional approaches of postdischarge SSI surveillance[44] include use of automated hospital discharge diagnosis codes, ambulatory diagnosis codes, and outpatient pharmacy dispensing data.[45-48] An example of computer programs for claims-based assessment of SSI after cardiac surgery is available.[49]

Once the research had been performed to conceive, develop, test, and evaluate the surrogate measure on a pilot basis, we would need to assess the feasibility of incorporating it into a production system that all health care organizations and/or payers could use. Data collection and aggregation of the surrogate measures would need to be examined in multicenter demonstration projects such as the one described earlier for SSIs.[35] These multicenter evaluations would also need to be capable of recalibrating surrogate measures because their predictive values would differ across organizations. Successively larger multicenter evaluations would be required before widescale adoption of a surrogate measure can be advanced.

Data from several sources—for example, different payers—may need to be combined to form a picture of a hospital's performance because any single payer is unlikely to have a sufficient volume of cases to allow accurate estimation of event rates. Although costs and logistics are major challenges to aligning computerized data that are currently available, progress is being made[50]; after systems to use these data are created, the costs of maintaining them is likely to be relatively low. Reexamination and recalibration of surrogate measures' accuracy and predictive value would be the continuing responsibility of the aggregating organization. Once a measure is developed and its accuracy assessed, an accrediting body such as The Joint Commission should use the information with an approach that is non-punitive and follows recent HICPAC recommendations.[40]

Comparing measures across organizations may give programs the signal to investigate a potential problem. However, high rates of surrogate measures would not necessarily prove that a problem exists. Comparisons should be used only as an initial guide for setting priorities for further investigation. In our example of the proportion of coronary artery bypass patients who receive at least nine days of antibiotics after surgery as a surrogate for SSI rates, organizations that have relatively high values for this measure may need to investigate the following questions:

- Are the data an accurate reflection of the hospital's experience, as determined by targeted record review?
- Is the number of procedures large enough to allow a precise enough estimate of the measure's performance?
- Does the organization's case mix differ substantially from those of other organizations and account for the high rate?
- Does the high proportion of patients receiving postoperative antibiotics represent patients with SSIs on appropriate therapy and why?
- Does the high proportion represent inappropriate antibiotic use?

If problems are identified, more detailed measurement may be desired for targeted high-risk or high-volume areas, such as those being developed in CDC's National Healthcare Safety Network.[51]

Development of surrogate measures would present challenges. We would need measures that have an acceptable balance between sensitivity and predictive value, but we should not insist on perfect sensitivity because underreporting is recognized as the biggest problem in current detection systems. Surrogate measures are much more likely to be useful for comparing organizations rather than individual clinicians, partly because case mix would be more difficult to control for individuals and because small sample sizes would mean that rates are unstable.

Outlier status of individual providers would be less informative and less appealing for committing the follow-up resources that would be required to assess the meaning of an unusual rate. Finally, surrogate measures would not be useful for monitoring very rare but catastrophic events such as nosocomial Creutzfeldt-Jakob disease or detecting the performance of the wrong procedure.

Conclusion

We cannot continue to rely on either voluntary, spontaneous reporting of health care–associated infections, and possibly other kinds of adverse events, or on individual expert assessment, to confirm every occurrence that suggests harm to a patient. The investment of resources and the potential for substantial additional improvement by this mechanism is limited. Many health care organizations claim that currently available measures are not relevant to care provided. Developing clinically relevant process or surrogate measures that clinicians would use to improve patient outcomes is essential. Objective and universal measures may be relevant not only to hospital-acquired infections but also to other health care–related adverse events that require substantial resources to identify. The development of process and surrogate measures would expand our use of electronic health information for a vital purpose: To improve patient safety. ■

References

1. Lee T.H., Meyer G.S., Brennan T.A.: A middle ground on public accountability. *N Eng J Med* 350:2409–2422, Jun. 3, 2003.

2. Institute of Medicine: *To Err Is Human: Building a Safer Health System.* Washington, DC: National Academy Press, 1999.

3. Altman D.E., Clancy C., Blendon R.J.: Improving patient safety—Five years after the IOM report. *N Engl J Med* 351:2041–2042, Nov. 11, 2004.

4. Gaynes R., Horan T.: Surveillance of nosocomial infections. In Mayhall C. (ed.): *Hospital Epidemiology and Infection Control.* Baltimore: Lippincott, William & Wilkins, 2004, pp. 1659–1702.

5. Wenzel R.P., Pfaller M.A.: Infection control: The premier quality assessment program in United States hospitals. *Am J Med* 91(3B):27S–31S, Sep. 16, 1991.

6. Stamm W.E., Weinstein R.A., Dixon R.E.: Comparison of endemic and epidemic nosocomial infections. *Am J Med* 170:393–397, Feb. 1981.

7. Haley R.W., et al.: The efficacy of infection surveillance and control programs in preventing nosocomial infections in U.S. hospitals. *Am J Epidemiol* 212:182–205, Feb. 1985.

8. Chorba T.L., et al.: Mandatory reporting of infectious diseases by clinicians. *JAMA* 262:3018–3026, Dec. 1, 1989.

9. Leape L.L.: Reporting of adverse events. *N Engl J Med* 347:1633–1638, Nov. 14, 2002.

10. Nguyen G.T., et al.: Status of infection surveillance and control programs in the United States, 1992–1996. Association for Professionals in Infection Control and Epidemiology, Inc. *Am J Infect Control* 28:392–400, Jun. 2000.

11. Bjerke N.B., et al.: Job analysis 1992: Infection control practitioner. *Am J Infect Control* 21:51–57, Apr. 1993.

12. O'Boyle C., Jackson M., Henly S.J.: Staffing requirements for infection control programs in US health care facilities: Delphi project. *Am J Infect Control* 30:321–333, Oct. 2002.

13. Emori T.G., et al.: National Nosocomial Infections Surveillance System (NNIS): Description of surveillance methods. *Am J Infect Control* 19:19–35, Feb. 1991.

14. Garner J.S., et al.: CDC definitions for nosocomial infections, 1988. *Am J Infect Control* 16:28–40, Jun. 1988.

15. Centers for Disease Control and Prevention: Monitoring hospital-acquired infections to promote patient safety—United States, 1990–1999. *MMWR* 49:149–53, Mar. 3, 2000.

16. Burke J.P.: Infection control: A problem for patient safety. *N Engl J Med* 348:651–656, Feb. 13, 2003.

17. Weigelt J.A., Dryer D., Haley R.W.: The necessity and efficiency of wound surveillance after discharge. *Arch Surg* 127:77–82, Jan. 1992.

18. Olson M.M., O'Connor M., Schwartz M.L.: Surgical wound infections: A 5 year prospective study of 20,193 wounds at the Minneapolis VA Medical Center. *Ann Surg* 199:253–259, Mar. 1984.

19. Zoutman D., et al.: Surgical wound infections occurring in day surgery patients. *Am J Infect Control* 18:277–282, Aug. 1990.

20. Salem R.J., Johnson J., Devitt P.: Short term metronidazole therapy contrasted with povidone iodine spray in the prevention of wound infection after appendectomy. *Br J Surg* 66:430–431, Jun. 1979.

21. Bates T., et al.: Prophylactic metronidazole in appendectomy: A controlled trial. *Br J Surg* 67:547–550, Jan. 1980.

22. Burns S.J., Dippe S.E.: Postoperative wound infections detected during hospitalization and after discharge in a community hospital. *Am J Infect Control* 10:60–65, May 1982.

23. Brown R.M., et al.: Surgical wound infections documented after hospital discharge. *Am J Infect Control* 15:54–58, Apr. 1987.

24. Rosendorf L.L., Octavio J., Estes J.P.: Effect of methods of postdischarge wound infection surveillance on reported infection rates. *Am J Infect Control* 11:226–229, Dec. 1983.

25. Polk F.B., et al.: Randomized clinical trial of perioperative cefazolin in preventing infection after hysterectomy. *Lancet* 1:437–441, Mar. 1, 1980.

26. Cruse P.J.E., Foord R.: A five-year prospective study of 23,649 wounds. *Arch Surg* 107:206–210, Aug. 1973.

27. Condon R.E., et al.: Effectiveness of a surgical wound surveillance program. *Arch Surg* 118:303–307, Mar. 1983.

28. Reimer K., Gleed C., Nicolle L.E.: The impact of postdischarge infection on surgical wound infection rates. *Infect Control* 8:237–240, Jun. 1987.

29. Manian F.A., Meyer L.: Comprehensive surveillance of surgical wound infections in outpatient and inpatient surgery. *Infect Control Hosp Epidemiol* 11:515–520, Jan. 1990.

30. Holbrook K.F., et al.: Automated postdischarge surveillance for postpartum and neonatal nosocomial infections. *Am J Med* 191 [Suppl. 3B]:125S–130S, Sep. 1991.

31. Hulton L.J., et al.: Effect of postdischarge surveillance on rates of infectious complications after cesarean section. *Am J Infect Control* 20:198–201, Aug. 1992.

32. Gaynes R.P.: Surgical site infections and the NNIS SSI Risk Index: Room for improvement. *Infect Control Hosp Epidemiol* 21:184–185, Mar. 2000.

33. Burke J.P.: Maximizing appropriate antibiotic prophylaxis for surgical patients: An update from LDS Hospital, Salt Lake City. *Clin Infect Dis* 33 (Suppl. 2):S78–S83, Sep. 2001.

34. Kerr E.A., et al.: Diabetes care quality in the veterans affairs health care system and commercial managed care: The TRIAD Study. *Ann Intern Med* 141:272–281, Aug. 17, 2004.

35. Yokoe D.S., et al.: Enhanced identification of postoperative infections among inpatients. *Emerg Infect Dis* 10:1924–1930, Nov. 2004.

36. Yokoe D.S., Platt R.: Surveillance for surgical site infections: The uses of antibiotic exposure. *Infect Control Hosp Epidemiol* 15:717–723, Nov. 1994.

37. Yokoe D.S., et al.: Use of antibiotic exposure to detect postoperative infections. *Infect Control Hosp Epidemiol* 19:317–322, May 1998.

38. Trick W.E., et al.: Computer algorithms to detect bloodstream infections. *Emerg Infect Dis* 10:1612–1620, Sep. 2004.

39. Yokoe D.S., et al.: Simplified surveillance for nosocomial bacteremias. *Infect Control Hosp Epidemiol* 19:657–660, Sep. 1998.

40. McKibben L.M., et al.: Guidance on Public Reporting of Healthcare-Associated Infections: Recommendations of the Healthcare Infection Control Practices Advisory Committee. *Infect Control Hosp Epidemiol* 26:5807, Jun. 2005.

This chapter first appeared in the February 2006 (Volume 32, Number 2, pages 95–101) issue of *The Joint Commission Journal on Quality and Patient Safety.*

Modifying the Universal Protocol for Effective Delivery of Perioperative Prophylactic Antibiotics

Gene N. Peterson, M.D.,
Ph.D., M.H.A.
Seth Hennessey, M.H.A.,
R.H.I.A.

Judy Westby, R.N.
Judith Canfield, R.N.
Diana Villaflor-Camagong,
M.H.A.

Effective delivery of perioperative antibiotics is one of the key measures in preventing surgical site infection.[1] Previous work has demonstrated that delivery of the appropriate antibiotic 0–60 minutes before surgery reduces the incidence of postoperative surgical site infections.[2] Successful delivery of antibiotics is being used as a marker of quality by the National Quality Forum,[3] is aligned with The Joint Commission's National Patient Safety Goal[4] of reducing the risk of health care–associated infections, and is being used by purchasing groups as a measure of effective care.[5]

About the Authors

Gene N. Peterson, M.D., Ph.D., M.H.A., is Associate Medical Director, and **Seth Hennessey, M.H.A., R.H.I.A.,** is Manager, Center for Clinical Excellence, University of Washington Medical Center, Seattle.

Judy Westby, R.N., is Nurse Manager, Surgical Services; **Judith Canfield, R.N.,** is Senior Associate Administrator, Surgical Services; and **Diana Villaflor-Camagong, M.H.A.,** is Infection Control Practitioner, Department of Epidemiology and Infection Control, University of Washington Medical Center.

Please address reprint requests to Gene N. Peterson, M.D., Ph.D., M.H.A., gpeterso@u.washington.edu.

The actual delivery of the perioperative antibiotics is a complex team task in the operating room (OR), involving antibiotic choice by the surgical team, choice of a time for delivery by the nursing and anesthesia team, and documentation of the delivery in the patient's medical record. This article describes improvement in our process of antibiotic delivery by leveraging our compliance with The Joint Commission's Universal Protocol for Preventing Wrong Site, Wrong Procedure, Wrong Person Surgery™ (Universal Protocol).[6]

Methods

SETTING
The University of Washington Medical Center (UWMC) participated in a Collaborative on Surgical Infection Prevention (CSIP) between March 2002 and April 2003, which was sponsored by the state of Washington's Medicare Quality Improvement Organization.

RESEARCH DESIGN
As suggested by the CSIP, we identified a small subset of all our surgical patients requiring perioperative antibiotics. We included only surgical procedures performed by three general surgeons and one orthopedic surgeon (champions), where the risk of postsurgical infection was high or the risk of infection was catastrophic. For this time period, a reporting measure was developed to track the organizationwide effectiveness of timely delivery of appropriate perioperative antibiotics. Data sources were the manual paper anesthesia record and the patient's paper medical chart. Automated drug administration records were not available. After Institutional Human Subjects Review, the data were abstracted by retrospective chart review.

Process Improvement
Figure 6-1 is a *p*-chart, with 1, 2, and 3 sigma upper and lower control limits, which shows the effectiveness of delivery of a perioperative antibiotic before surgery. Antibiotics were scored as appropriately delivered if a perioperative prophylactic antibiotic was given in the perioperative period by either the nursing or anesthesia staff.

Between July 2002 and April 2003, little improvement was made through standard quality improvement techniques of education, signage, and encouragement. On September 1, 2003, the UWMC made an institutional change in the formal Universal Protocol recommendations by adding a step to the work process that included a question on whether the perioperative antibiotics had been or are being given (*see* Table 6-1). The anesthesia team, nursing team, and surgical team all confirmed the administration of antibiotics, if indicated, for the procedure. To measure the effectiveness of this intervention, we used the same subset of surgical patients identified during our CSIP, which had ended three months earlier.

FIGURE 6-1. Delivery of Appropriate Antibiotic Before Surgery

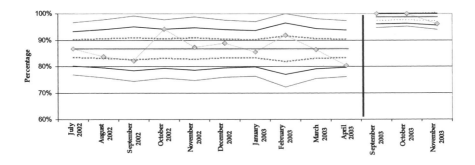

The mean value and control limits (1 [dashed line], 2 [black line], and 3 [grey line] sigma) are shown; for the September 2003–November 2003 period, the control limits were all 100%. The July 2002–April 2003 data represent an average of 82 observations per month, and the September 2003–November 2003 data represent an average of 71 observations per month. The vertical line represents the intervention.

Source: Authors.

Results

As shown in the *p*-chart (Figure 6-1, above), there was a significant improvement in delivery of the perioperative antibiotics for the months September to November 2003. The preintervention baseline of 823 patients (86% effectiveness) and postintervention delivery rates of 212 patients (98% effectiveness) are significantly different ($p < .01$) using the *z*-test of proportions.

Discussion

Delivery of perioperative antibiotics is an OR task that requires cooperation between the surgeon, who typically requests the antibiotics, and the anesthesia and surgical nursing teams, who are usually responsible for delivery of the drugs. Unfortunately, the interval for antibiotic delivery before surgical incision is the busiest time for the nursing and anesthesia staff, who are involved in obtaining all the necessary equipment and supplies for the surgery, complying with all the required consent and verification procedures, and inducing anesthesia for the surgery itself.

TABLE 6-1. Final Perioperative Safety Check List (FPSCL)

- Circulating R.N. coordinates the FPSCL.
- Anesthesia Representative reads out loud the patient's name and hospital number from their ID wristband.
- Circulating R.N. and Surgical Representative confirm that the name and hospital number agree with those on the patient's consent form.
- Circulating R.N. reads the consent out loud, including the side of surgery.
- Surgical Representative verifies that the correct side/site is marked and that it will be visible following prepping and draping for surgery.
- Circulating R.N. confirms with the Anesthesia Representative that the antibiotics have been/are being given, except in cases where cultures are needed before giving antibiotics.*
- Circulating R.N. and Surgical Representative verify that the x-rays (if present) are the same side as the patient's consent.
- Circulating R.N. asks, "Any other concerns?" If none, proceed with case.

* Check for antibiotics.

Source: Authors.

Before modifying the Universal Protocol our organization tried education of the anesthesia providers regarding the value of perioperative antibiotics, signage reminders in the OR room and holding areas, and verbal and e-mail reminders to all involved in the process. Yet, as is evident from Figure 1, there was little or no improvement in our antibiotic delivery performance.

We in fact may have been operating at our best level of 10^{-1}–10^{-2} reliability, depending only on the anesthesia provider to deliver the antibiotic by memory and best effort.[7] By modifying the Universal Protocol we were able to have the entire team focus on not only the verification of the patient identification, surgical site, and procedure but also the selection and delivery of the perioperative antibiotic. In addition to confirming that we had the right patient for the right surgery on the right site, we also confirmed that we gave the patient the appropriate antibiotic. Use of the checklist improved an important process and, hopefully, will lead us to further improvements in our communication and team coordination.[8]

As in any quality improvement project there are limitations to what we can glean from the data. We attribute this improvement to the change in process of delivering antibiotics, but it could actually represent an improvement in documentation or changes in process during the summer of 2003 between the end of the CSIP and our intervention. To the best knowledge of the investigators, there were few changes in the methods of perioperative antibiotic delivery during the months of May 2003 to August 2003, although we do not have performance data for that period. We considered the baseline we had previously established as adequate to determine if our intervention worked, and we chose not to repeat data collection and delay the intervention's implementation. We have data from September 2003 to November 2003 to support the final verification intervention but cannot document the intervention's sustainability. We have implemented this process improvement throughout the entire population at UWMC and encourage its replication at other organizations. ■

References

1. Mangram A.J., et al.: Guideline for Prevention of Surgical Site Infection 1999. *Infect Control Hosp Epidemiol* 20:250–278, Apr. 1999.

2. Burke J.P.: Infection control: A problem for patient safety. *N Engl J Med* 348:651–656, Feb. 13, 2003.

3. National Quality Forum: *Safe Practices for Better Healthcare.* http://www.qualityforum.org/txsafeexecsumm+order6-8-03PUBLIC.pdf (accessed Dec. 9, 2005).

4. The Joint Commission: *2005 Hospitals' National Patient Safety Goals.* http://www.jcaho.org/accredited+organizations/patient+safety/05+npsg/05_npsg_hap.htm (accessed Dec. 9, 2005).

5. The Leapfrog Group: *The Leapfrog Group Hospital Quality and Survey.* https://leapfrog.medstat.com/pdf/Final.pdf (accessed Dec. 9, 2005).

6. The Joint Commission: *Universal Protocol for Preventing Wrong Site, Wrong Procedure, Wrong Person Surgery™.* http://www.jcaho.org/accredited+organizations/patient+safety/universal+protocol/wss_universal+protocol.htm (accessed Dec. 9, 2005).

7. Amalberti R., et al.: Five system barriers to achieving ultrasafe health care *Ann Intern Med* 142:756–764, May 3, 2005.

8. Sexton, J.B., Thomas, E.J., Helmreich, R.L.: Error, stress and teamwork in medicine and aviation: Cross sectional surveys. *BMJ* 320:745–749, Mar. 18, 2000.

This chapter first appeared in the February 2006 (Volume 32, Number 2, pages 92–94) issue of *The Joint Commission Journal on Quality and Patient Safety.*

SECTION 2

Infection Prevention and Control Practice

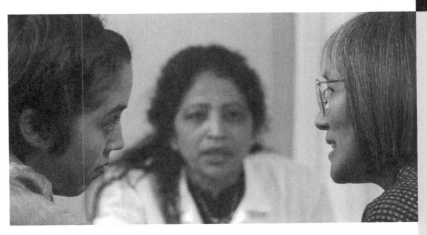

Private Rooms and the Environment of Care: Organizations Recognizing the Safety and Privacy Benefits of Single-Patient Rooms

ENVIRONMENT

The growing trend toward private patient rooms picked up speed in June 2006, when the American Institute of Architects (AIA) and the Facility Guidelines Institute (FGI) released new design standards for health care facilities. The 2006 edition of *Guidelines for Design and Construction of Hospital and Health Care Facilities* adopts single-bed rooms as a "minimum standard" for new hospital construction. While these guidelines do not apply to all hospitals (and are not now required by Joint Commission standards), they reflect the growing appreciation of how private rooms can positively affect the environment of care.

"While competition for patients is one factor driving this trend, the move toward private rooms is based solidly on care-related benefits," says John Fishbeck, R.A., associate director in the Division of Standards and Survey Methods, The Joint Commission. "Private rooms contribute significantly to patient safety and privacy and appear to have a positive impact on care outcomes."

Safety Issues

Experts in health care environmental design point to several clinical benefits of private patient rooms. Joseph G. Sprague, F.A.I.A., F.A.C.H.A., served as the chair of the committee that produced the new AIA/FGI Guidelines. He says one major advantage of private room design is better infection control. "In a multibed room, caregivers can spread infections by handling common elements—curtains, computer terminals, anything in the room," he says. "*The Guidelines* committee found that private rooms offer a substantial potential to reduce these cross-infections." Given that 5 to 10% of hospital inpatients acquire health care–associated infections (*see* Chapter 11, "National Data Report: Hospital Infection Reporting Guidelines," pages 111–116), the desirability of private rooms becomes all the more apparent.

Sprague, who serves as president of the FGI, is also senior vice president, director of health facilities, for HKS, Inc., an architectural firm headquartered in Dallas. He says the new private room recommendation reflects the consensus of a multidisciplinary group of experts, including physicians, nurses, facilities engineers, and architects. "One of the major issues the committee looked at was medical errors, especially errors that can result when caregivers confuse patient identities," he says. "When more than one patient is in a room, there is a substantial potential for the administration of a wrong medication or a wrong therapy." Meal mix-ups pose another risk, especially in the case of a patient on a strictly prescribed diet. "It's pretty clear that if there is only one patient in a room, there will be no problem with these kinds of mistakes," he says. "The guidelines committee believes that reducing these opportunities contributes to a safer environment for patients."

One of the main reasons private rooms are potentially safer is that they reduce the need for patient transfers. In a multibed environment, supervisors must frequently shift patients to different rooms to accommodate changes in acuity, avoid different gender pairings, and address problems such as behavior issues. These transfers can be another cause of the confusion that leads to wrong-meal, wrong-therapy, and wrong-medication errors. They also seemingly increase the potential for patient falls and staff injuries.

A literature review sponsored by the FGI revealed mixed evidence on the impact of private rooms on patient falls.[1] For patients who need constant supervision, multibed rooms that are potentially easier for staff to monitor could provide better support for fall prevention. On the other hand, private rooms can more easily accommodate family members. If family members are more likely to be on hand to monitor patients and help them move about, this could reduce the incidence of patient falls.

Superior Privacy

Of course, one of the main advantages of single-bed rooms is patient privacy. "No one would go to a hotel and have a roommate, yet we expect people to have a

SECTION 2
ENVIRONMENT

CHAPTER 7: Private Rooms and the Environment of Care:
Organizations Recognizing the Safety and Privacy Benefits
of Single-Patient Rooms

roommate in the hospital," says Dale Woodin, deputy executive director of the American Society for Healthcare Engineering (ASHE). "Probably the biggest benefit of the single-bed room is the opportunity to have a private environment."

Practically speaking, private rooms offer patients the ability to rest better and get more undisturbed sleep. Sprague says the AIA/FGI *Guidelines* committee considered personal control to be a key issue: "Private room design gives the patient control over his or her environment." This can translate into a greater sense of dignity, a feeling that is easily lost in a hospital environment. It also supports important clinical communication. "Private rooms allow patients to communicate freely and openly with doctors, nurses, or therapists with no hesitancy that they might be overheard," says Sprague. The private environment also enables family members to take a more positive role in discussions and is a better environment for interactions with clergy. Sprague believes private rooms are essential to compliance with privacy regulations. "The only way to comply with the Health Insurance Portability and Accountability Act of 1996 is with private rooms—there is no way to be in compliance in a multibed setting."

Overall, single-bed rooms appear to have a positive impact on clinical outcomes. "The consensus of the guidelines committee was that private rooms substantially reduce the length of stay for patients," says Sprague. He notes that the therapeutic value of the private environment may speed recovery: "These patients are getting to lower acuity levels and out of the hospital more quickly."

Going All-Private

For many hospitals, the private room advantage is so compelling that they plan to phase out multipatient rooms altogether. That is the vision of facilities planners at Children's Medical Center Dallas, a nonprofit pediatric hospital licensed for 406 beds. According to Louis Saksen, AIA, the medical center's vice president for facilities, Children's stopped building double rooms in the late 1990s. By 2012, he says, there will be no multibed rooms left in the organization.

"Our primary impetus in going to all private rooms is patient safety," says Saksen, citing advantages in infection control, noise, and medication and dietary errors. He notes that caregivers at Children's prefer the private room arrangement. "Physicians and nurses find it easier to deliver care when there are not two patients in a room," he says. "Certainly from a patient privacy standpoint, it is a lot easier: Caregivers can talk to the patient and the patient's family without the concern of being overheard."

Saksen also notes that private rooms do away with the conflicts that arise when an extended family is visiting one patient in a multibed room and the other patient is alone. "I don't know how to quantify it, but the level of anxiety our patients experience is definitely reduced by not having another patient and that patient's family members and caregivers in the room." One of the most positive aspects of private room design is that it can enable parents to stay overnight. "In our new construction, we are including enough room for two parents—or a parent and a sibling—to stay in the hospital with the patient," he says. "For these little kids, this is very, very important."

Do private rooms cause problems with surge capacity? Saksen says that Children's worked this possibility into its plans. "In the rooms we converted from double to single, we left the head walls in place, so all we have to do to increase capacity is move another bed back in," he says. "We retained the ability to flex up during an emergency."

Still Room for Multibeds

Not everyone believes private rooms should be mandatory for hospitals. According to Woodin, ASHE's position is that decisions about private versus shared rooms should be made locally: "We feel that private rooms represent a great best practice, but the choice belongs to the hospital."

Joseph Sprague says the new AIA/FGI *Guidelines* recognize that in certain circumstances, multipatient rooms are appropriate. "The *Guidelines* give hospital planners the flexibility and opportunity to design multibed rooms when they can demonstrate to the authorities that it is necessary," he says.

For many hospitals, a compelling reason to build multibed rooms might be serious space constraints. For example, private rooms could be impractical for an urban high-rise hospital with a strictly limited footprint. Other valid reasons could be related to community demographics. "In a rural hospital with very limited staff, there may not be enough nurses to cover a unit that is all private rooms," says

SECTION 2
ENVIRONMENT

CHAPTER 7: Private Rooms and the Environment of Care:
Organizations Recognizing the Safety and Privacy Benefits
of Single-Patient Rooms

Sprague. Another possible rationale for choosing multibed rooms is therapeutic value. According to Sprague, some argue that orthopedic patients, who have longer lengths of stay, progress more satisfactorily when they have roommates. Woodin says the same might also apply to behavioral health and geriatric patients.

What if a health care organization simply cannot afford to include private rooms in new construction? Sprague says the new AIA/FGI *Guidelines* recognize economics as a potentially valid argument against single-bed rooms, but he notes that the long-term savings from private rooms can balance out the higher initial investment. "While it may take a bit more in capital dollars to build an all-private facility—the speculation is 5% to 15%, depending on whom you talk to—the reduction in operational costs is potentially significant." Studies cited in the FGI–sponsored literature review identify several reasons private room operating costs are lower, including higher bed occupancy rates and lower costs associated with patient transfers.[1]

Environment Option

As noted previously, The Joint Commission does not now require hospitals to design new construction with private rooms. (Standard EC.8.30, element of performance 1, currently references the 2001 edition of the *Guidelines*, not the new 2006 edition.) Still, Joint Commission experts point out that the benefits of private room design mesh with the broad goals of the Management of the Environment of Care (EC) standards.

According to the overview in the EC chapter of the 2007 *Comprehensive Accreditation Manual for Hospitals: The Official Handbook*, design elements such as space size, configuration, and layout should "create safe, welcoming, and comfortable environments that support and maintain patient dignity and personhood, allow ease of interaction, reduce stressors, and encourage family participation in the delivery of care." John Fishbeck of The Joint Commission notes that private rooms can be effective at advancing these objectives. He adds that single-bed design also supports compliance with several National Patient Safety Goals, particularly those related to patient identification, infection, fall prevention, and patient and family involvement.

"Given the many clinical, safety, and privacy advantages of private rooms," says Fishbeck, "health care leaders are encouraged to seriously consider this design option when planning for the environment of care." ■

Reference

1. American Institute of Architects: *The Use of Single Patient Rooms Versus Multiple Occupancy Rooms in Acute Care Environments.* http://www.aia.org/SiteObjects/files/ 05_Pilot_Study_on_Assessment.pdf (accessed Jan. 25, 2007).

This chapter is modified from its original form in the newsletter *Environment of Care News®*, Volume 9, Number 8, August 2006, pp. 1–3, for inclusion in this book.

Building Contractor Awareness: One Hospital Uses a Handbook to Help Educate Construction Workers

ENVIRONMENT

On any given day in a hospital, several construction projects can be under way at one time. These projects can be minimally invasive, such as installing a new piece of equipment, or they can be quite extensive, such as putting on a new wing or addition. Depending on the project, one or more contractors may be entering and exiting the building at various hours of the day and night. They may bring in equipment, remove waste, or create dust. The work may be noisy and can add confusion to a place that is already both complex and hectic.

To help ensure open two-way communication between hospital staff and contractors, St. Joseph Hospital in Orange, California, created a contractor handbook. This document is given to any contractor doing work in the facility. The handbook provides clearly written information on the hospital's policies regarding fire safety, security, conduct, smoking, hazardous materials disposal, infection control, patient privacy, and many more issues. (*See* the handbook's table of contents in Figure 8-1, page 99) It also provides phone numbers for key hospital staff members, such as the director of plant services, safety officer, and infection control officer. The handbook includes copies of forms and checklists, which the contractor should use in conjunction with hospital staff to assess interim life safety measures, infection control measures, and so forth.

Why Create the Handbook?

Several years ago, staff members at St. Joseph began to notice some safety issues related to construction work. "I caught one plumber soldering a pipe in the ceiling without a fire extinguisher nearby," says Jim Veler, director of plant services for St.

Joseph Hospital. "Our IC (infection control) specialist observed some contractors carrying a pipe down a hallway past patient rooms. It was clear we needed to do something to educate contractors about the safety requirements of our hospital."

To address the issue, the organization began to outline the information that contractors needed to maintain a safe environment. "We wanted all individuals working in our facility to be aware of evacuation procedures, telephone numbers, parking requirements, fire safety issues, and infection control issues. Our hospital has a dress code, a smoking policy, and expects proper conduct from individuals working in the facility. When we began to list all the information contractors needed to know, it became obvious that we needed a total contractor's handbook," says Veler.

Creating the Handbook

To create the handbook, St. Joseph used a multidisciplinary approach. Representatives from the infection control, security, construction, and plant services departments, as well as the safety officer and ergonomics officer all provided input regarding the content of the handbook. The local fire inspector also reviewed it. "Our organization uses a few large contractors, and we solicited their feedback on the handbook as well," says Veler. When input was received and the document created, the handbook was reviewed and approved by the organization's environment of care (EC) committee. "While it was challenging to incorporate everyone's feedback, it was important that the handbook be comprehensive yet easily understood by a contractor," says Cindy Thurman, work control coordinator of plant services for St. Joseph Hospital.

How It Works

Before a contractor can start work at St. Joseph Hospital, he or she must obtain a permit from the plant operations department, unless the plant operations department deems a permit unnecessary. (For example, if the contractor is delivering new bedside tables, a permit is not necessary.) To receive a permit, the contractor must review the contractor handbook and understand its contents. The contractor must then sign the handbook to indicate that he or she has reviewed the document and is familiar with it.

The plant operations department is responsible for training contractors to be compliant with the handbook. "We generally use the same contractors for most of

FIGURE 8-1. St. Joseph's Contractor's Handbook Table of Contents

Table of Contents Page

Table of Contents Page

SIGNATURE* ____________________ Date:__________

COMPANY NAME* ____________________

*My signature verifies that I have read the Contractor's Handbook, am familiar with its contents, and am aware of the appropriate resources for concerns related to health and safety on the job, have received and will strictly adhere to St. Joseph's Infection Control and Wall & Floor Penetration Policies and Procedures. This handbook will be reviewed with all subcontractors.

This is an example of what one organization is doing to help educate construction contractors.

Source: St. Joseph Hospital.

our construction projects, so we train them on the handbook and require them to train any subcontractors they use," says Veler.

To ensure compliance with the handbook, hospital staff must sign off on a job before a contractor is paid. "Our hospital is divided into zones, and each zone has a mechanic who is in charge of inspecting the work covered by a permit and verifying that work was conducted appropriately," says Veler.

In addition, the organization has a policy allowing any member of plant services, security, or hospital management to stop a contractor and ask to see his or her work permit. If the contractor cannot provide the permit, the hospital staff should contact plant services immediately to resolve the issue.

Benefits of the Handbook

"Doing construction work in a hospital is not the same as doing work in an apartment complex or office building, and the handbook helps educate contractors on that fact. They are working around potentially compromised individuals, and they need to monitor their work habits accordingly," says Veler. "The handbook helps make contractors accountable and ensures that every step of a project is looked at carefully."

The handbook also provides an opportunity to document the work being done in the hospital. "Because all contractors must sign the handbook before receiving a permit, we can track all the work occurring in the facility and quickly identify any potential issues that need attention," says Veler.

A Living Document

To ensure that the handbook is current, St. Joseph reviews it every year. "We need to make sure that the handbook addresses all applicable standards and regulatory requirements and is in line with hospital policy. Since standards, regulations, and policies change, our handbook must change along with them," says Thurman. By reviewing the handbook frequently, the organization can help make sure it is providing the safest possible environment for patients and staff.

This chapter is modified from its original form in the newsletter *Environment of Care News*, Volume 9, Number 4, April 2006, pp. 6–11 for inclusion in this book.

Preparing for a Pandemic: Infection Control Experts Discuss Avian Flu— and Not "Whether" but "When"

ENVIRONMENT

"How far do infected people fly? All over the world," says Nancy Kupka, D.N.Sc., M.P.H., R.N., project director, Department of Standards and Survey Methods, The Joint Commission. "So an infected person may feel fine and get on a plane, taking the flu almost anywhere in the world."

Kupka goes on to caution about the need to be prepared for an influx of infectious patients, as described in Joint Commission Standards EC.4.10–EC.4.20 and IC.6.10. And the flu to which she refers isn't just the yearly human flu that afflicts the United States every winter but a relatively new subtype of influenza A viruses known as H5N1—otherwise referred to as "avian flu." Since it surfaced in southern China in 1997, this virus has become stronger and deadlier, killing not just geese and ducks but domesticated chickens and now humans. What concerns public health officials most is the deadly nature of the virus. As of January 12, 2007, about 265 people were known to have contracted it. Of those, avian flu killed 159 people, or 60%.[1] One of the most notorious flu pandemics before avian flu, the Spanish flu pandemic of 1918, killed only 1% to 2% of its victims.

It has been 37 years since the last pandemic (for more historical detail, *see* Figure 9-1), and many scientists believe that it's only a matter of time until the next influenza pandemic, aided in part by the facility of air travel around the world. Although no one knows how severe the next pandemic will be, studies suggest that its effect in the United States could be disastrous. If efforts to develop an effective vaccine are unsuccessful, estimates are that a medium-level pandemic here could cause 89,000 to 207,000 deaths, between 314,000 and 734,000 hospitalizations, 18 to 42 million

---

FIGURE 9-1. Short History of Influenza Pandemics

The first known influenza pandemic occurred between 1889 and 1890 and killed an estimated 1 million people throughout Europe and Asia. In the twentieth century, flu pandemics have occurred with disturbing regularity:

→ 1918–1919—Spanish flu killed more than 675,000 people in the United States and as many as 50 million people worldwide in 18 months. Many people died within the first few days after infection, and others died of complications later. Nearly half of those who died were young, healthy adults.

→ 1957–1958—Asian flu caused about 70,000 deaths in the United States. First identified in China in late February 1957, the Asian flu spread to the United States by June 1957.

→ 1968–1969—Hong Kong flu resulted in about 34,000 deaths in the United States. The virus was first detected in Hong Kong in early 1968 and spread to the United States later that year. Various strains of this virus still circulate today.

Source: Portions of this figure were adapted from U.S. Department of Health and Human Services: *Pandemics and Pandemic Threats Since 1900,* available online at http://www.pandemicflu.gov/general/historicaloverview.html (accessed Jan. 16, 2007).

---

outpatient visits, and the sickening of another 20 to 47 million people. Between 15% and 35% of the U.S. population could be affected by an influenza pandemic, and the economic impact could range from $71.3 billion to $166.5 billion.[2]

The Clinical Side

Tim Uyeki, M.D., M.P.H., is a medical epidemiologist in the influenza branch of the Centers for Disease Control and Prevention (CDC) in Washington, D.C. "There have been sporadic cases of avian-to-human transmission of avian influenza (H5N1) viruses, generally through direct handling of infected poultry. There have been a few rare cases of limited person-to-person transmission in which an infected person probably transmitted the flu to a close contact," he reports. "But there's no evidence of sustained person-to-person transmission of H5N1 viruses."

Uyeki predicts that if this virus acquires the ability to spread from person to person in a sustained manner, it will trigger a global pandemic. "Because it's a new

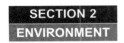

SECTION 2
ENVIRONMENT

CHAPTER 9: Preparing for a Pandemic: Infection
Control Experts Discuss Avian Flu—
and Not "Whether" but "When"

subtype of influenza A viruses that has never before circulated among people, previous vaccinations for other human flu strains wouldn't protect people, and we have acquired no immunity."

Uyeki maintains that although human flu viruses can cause severe complications and even death, the inflammatory response from H5N1 avian flu is "very abnormal" and far more severe than human flu viruses.

"In a year with a severe outbreak of human flu, we might have a great many sick people but still have many healthy caregivers because of vaccine," says Louise Kuhny, R.N., M.P.H., associate director, Standards Interpretation Group, The Joint Commission. "But because no one has any immunity to avian flu and there is currently no vaccine, the concern is that we could have a larger group of sick people and not enough health care workers to care for them."

What's Different This Time

The CDC warns that there are several key differences between influenza pandemics and many of the threats for which public health and the health care systems are currently planning. First, a pandemic would last much longer than most other emergency events and might include waves of influenza activity separated by months. Second, the number of health care workers and first responders available to work would likely be reduced because they'd be at risk of illness through exposure in the community and in health care settings. Some might have to miss work to care for ill family members. Third, resources in many locations could be limited because of how widespread an influenza pandemic would be.

Preparing for an Influx of Infectious Patients

When the possibility of a pandemic escalates from "whether" to "when" and then to "now," health care facilities must be ready for an influx of infectious patients in need of treatment. Most important in protecting staff and patients is recognizing the likelihood that avian flu, like human flu, is spread via droplets. For that reason, the CDC recommends standard precautions plus droplet precautions for known flu strains. However, the CDC also recommends additional precautions for health care workers involved in the care of avian flu patients.

The CDC urges facilities to pay particularly close attention to patients who've traveled in the previous 10 days to countries with avian flu activity and who are hospitalized with a severe febrile respiratory illness. In managing these patients, health care facilities should use isolation precautions identical to those recommended for patients with known severe acute respiratory syndrome, which are as follows:

- Pay careful attention to hand hygiene before and after all patient contact or contact with items potentially contaminated with respiratory secretions.
- Use gloves and gown for all patient contact.
- Use dedicated equipment such as stethoscopes, disposable blood pressure cuffs, disposable thermometers, and so on.
- Wear goggles or face shields within three feet of the patient.
- Place the patient in an airborne isolation room with monitored negative air pressure in relation to the corridor. The room should have 6 to 12 air changes per hour and should exhaust air directly to the outside or have recirculated air filtered by a high-efficiency particulate air (HEPA) filter. If an airborne isolation room isn't available, contact the health care facility engineer to assist or use portable HEPA filters (*see* "Environmental Infection Control Guidelines" at http://www.cdc.gov/ncidod/hip/enviro/guide.htm) to augment the number of air changes per hour.
- When entering the room, use a fit-tested respirator, at least as protective as a NIOSH–approved N-95 disposable filtering face-piece respirator.

Using Joint Commission Standards to Stay Ready

The Joint Commission's Kupka and Kuhny also recommend adhering to Standards IC.6.10 on infection control and EC.4.10–EC.4.20 on emergency management. Among the issues to be considered should be the following:

- Staying current on the local, national, and worldwide situation
- Staying in touch with local public health authorities via phone, fax, and e-mail
- Working with other hospitals in the area during an outbreak
- Determining whether to remain open to new patients

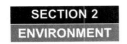

CHAPTER 9: Preparing for a Pandemic: Infection
Control Experts Discuss Avian Flu—
and Not "Whether" but "When"

- Preparing for an influx of infected patients
- Training staff members on the basics of infection control to protect themselves and patients
- Deciding whether to hold patients in the hospital for longer than normal rather than sending them to a home environment that may be infected
- Keeping staff members, physicians, and pharmacists informed on the latest news and hospital conditions and directives
- Alerting the purchasing department to replenish supplies, particularly personal protective equipment
- Putting admitting, housekeeping, and maintenance departments on alert

"Staying on top of infection control and environment of care issues can help organizations be prepared for the possibility of a pandemic," concludes Kupka. ■

References

1. World Health Association: *Cumulative Number of Confirmed Human Cases of Avian Influenza A/(H5N1) Reported to WHO.* http://www.who.int/csr/disease/avian_influenza/country/cases_table_2007_01_12/en/index.html (accessed Jan. 16, 2007).

2. Meltzer M.I., Cox N.J., Fukuda K.: The economic impact of pandemic influenza in the United States: Priorities for intervention. *Emerg Infect Dis* 5:659–671, Sep.–Oct. 1999.

This chapter is modified from its original form in the newsletter *Environment of Care News,* Volume 9, Number 1, January 2006, pp. 10–11 for inclusion in this book.

Surgical Care Infection Prevention Data Are Collected to Reduce Incidence of Surgical Complications

DATA

The Surgical Care Improvement Project (SCIP), a national quality partnership of 10 national organizations, including The Joint Commission, continues working toward its ultimate goal of reducing the incidence of surgical complications by 25% by 2010 by collecting surgical infection data from U.S. hospitals.

Accredited hospitals that elect to gather and submit data to The Joint Commission to meet their ORYX® (*see* http://www.jointcommission.org/AccreditationPrograms/Hospitals/ORYX/ for details) performance measurement requirements must report data on three SCIP infection measures (SCIP-1, SCIP-2, and SCIP-3) and two venous thromboembolism (VTE) measures (VTE-1 and VTE-2). Those data are made available to the public on The Joint Commission's Quality Check® Web site. Over time, The Joint Commission will likely require additional SCIP measures to be reported (*see* Figure 10-1 for complete list).

Overall (separate of The Joint Commission's accreditation process), participation in the SCIP involves the following:

- Collecting and submitting data on the measures
- Participating in monthly conference calls and sharing best practices and implementation strategies
- Making system changes based on quality improvement data

For more information on SCIP, including information on how to submit data not required by The Joint Commission, go to the Center for Medicare & Medicaid Services' MedQIC Web site at http://www.medqic.org. ■

FIGURE 10-1. Surgical Care Infection Prevention (SCIP) Process and Outcome Measures

Note: Measures in bold are those currently reported to The Joint Commission.

Infection (INF)

- **SCIP INF 1: Prophylactic antibiotic received within one hour prior to surgical incision***
  - **SCIP-INF-1a**   **Overall Rate**
  - **SCIP-INF-1b**   **Coronary Artery Bypass Graft**
  - **SCIP-INF-1c**   **Cardiac Surgery**
  - **SCIP-INF-1d**   **Hip Arthroplasty**
  - **SCIP-INF-1e**   **Knee Arthroplasty**
  - **SCIP-INF-1f**   **Colon Surgery**
  - **SCIP-INF-1g**   **Hysterectomy**
  - **SCIP-INF-1h**   **Vascular Surgery**

- **SCIP INF 2: Prophylactic antibiotic selection for surgical patients***
  - **SCIP-INF-2a**   **Overall Rate**
  - **SCIP-INF-2b**   **Coronary Artery Bypass Graft**
  - **SCIP-INF-2c**   **Cardiac Surgery**
  - **SCIP-INF-2d**   **Hip Arthroplasty**
  - **SCIP-INF-2e**   **Knee Arthroplasty**
  - **SCIP-INF-2f**   **Colon Surgery**
  - **SCIP-INF-2g**   **Hysterectomy**
  - **SCIP-INF-2h**   **Vascular Surgery**

- **SCIP INF 3: Prophylactic antibiotic discontinued within 24 hours after surgery end time (48 hours for cardiac patients)***
  - **SCIP-INF-3a**   **Overall Rate**
  - **SCIP-INF-3b**   **Coronary Artery Bypass Graft**
  - **SCIP-INF-3c**   **Cardiac Surgery**
  - **SCIP-INF-3d**   **Hip Arthroplasty**
  - **SCIP-INF-3e**   **Knee Arthroplasty**
  - **SCIP-INF-3f**   **Colon Surgery**
  - **SCIP-INF-3g**   **Hysterectomy**
  - **SCIP-INF-3h**   **Vascular Surgery**

- SCIP INF 4: Cardiac surgery patients with controlled 6 A.M. postoperative serum glucose

- SCIP INF 5: Postoperative wound infection diagnosed during index hospitalization (Outcome)

- SCIP INF 6: Surgery patients with appropriate hair removal

- SCIP INF 7: Colorectal surgery patients with immediate postoperative normothermia

*This measure, although part of SCIP program, is stratified by seven surgical procedure groups, with each surgical procedure group reported as a unique measure by The Joint Commission.

continued on page 109

FIGURE 10-1. Surgical Care Infection Prevention (SCIP) Process
and Outcome Measures, *continued*

Cardiac (CARD)
- SCIP CARD 1: Noncardiac vascular surgery patients with evidence of coronary artery disease who received beta-blockers during the preoperative period
- SCIP CARD 2: Surgery patients on a beta-blocker prior to arrival who received a beta-blocker during the preoperative period
- SCIP CARD 3: Intra- or postoperative acute myocardial infarction diagnosed during index hospitalization and within 30 days of surgery (Outcome)

Venous thromboembolism (VTE)
- **SCIP VTE 1: Surgery patients with recommended venous thromboembolism prophylaxis ordered**
- **SCIP VTE 2: Surgery patients who received appropriate venous thromboembolism prophylaxis within 24 hours prior to surgery to 24 hours after surgery**
- SCIP VTE 3: Intra- or postoperative pulmonary embolism diagnosed during index hospitalization and within 30 days of surgery (Outcome)
- SCIP VTE 4: Intra- or postoperative deep vein thrombosis diagnosed during index hospitalization and within 30 days of surgery (Outcome)

Respiratory (RESP)
- SCIP RESP 1: Number of days ventilated surgery patients had documentation of the head of the bed being elevated from recovery end date (day zero) through postoperative day seven.
- SCIP RESP 2: Patients diagnosed with postoperative ventilator-associated pneumonia during index hospitalization (Outcome)
- SCIP RESP 3: Number of days ventilated surgery patients had documentation of stress ulcer disease prophylaxis from recovery end date (day zero) through postoperative day seven.
- SCIP RESP 4: Surgery patients whose medical record contained an order for a ventilator weaning program (protocol or clinical pathway)

Other Measures
- SCIP Global 1: Mortality within 30 days of surgery
- SCIP Global 2: Readmission within 30 days of surgery
- VA 1: Proportion of permanent hospital end-stage renal disease vascular access procedures that are autogenous arteriovenous fistulas

Source: Modified from materials provided by the Quality Improvement Organization Program of Centers for Medicare & Medicaid Services at http://www.medqic.org/dcs/ContentServer?cid=1136495755695&pagename=Medqic%2FOtherResource%2FOtherResourcesTemplate&c=OtherResource.

This chapter is modified from its original form in the newsletter *The Joint Commission Benchmark*®, Volume 8, Number 2, March/April 2006, p. 6 for inclusion in this book. Portions of this chapter were also modified from materials provided by the Quality Improvement Organization Program of the Centers for Medicare & Medicaid Services at http://www.medqic.org/dcs/ContentServer? cid=1136495755695&pagename=Medqic%2FOtherResource%2FOtherResources Template&c=OtherResource.

National Data Report: Hospital Infection Reporting Guidelines

DATA

What is the most common complication affecting hospitalized patients? What accounts for an estimated 90,000 deaths and approximately $4.5 billion in health care costs[1] each year? The answer to both questions is hospital-acquired infections, also known as health care–associated infections (HAIs). The bad news is that between 5% and 10% of inpatients acquire one or more infections during a hospital stay; the good news is that some experts believe that at least 20% to 30% of these infections can be prevented,[2] and recent studies suggest even higher prevention rates.[3] Stakeholders—including health care providers, regulators, insurers, professional associations, patient advocacy groups, and the general public—are looking for answers to the challenge of reducing infection rates and improving prevention practices.

One of the solutions proposed by several stakeholder groups is the public disclosure of hospital infection rates. The rationale is twofold: First, the information should help patients, employers, and insurers make more informed decisions about where to go for safer care; second, the competition will force hospitals to bring infection control and prevention practices up to par. Currently, 6 states (Florida, Illinois, Missouri, New York, Pennsylvania, and Virginia) have passed legislation requiring hospitals to publicly report HAI rates, and more than 30 others have legislation pending. Nevada requires reporting to the state, but the results are not available to the public.

Critics of mandatory public reporting point to the lack of standardization in data collection and reporting methods as major barriers to the usefulness of this strategy. Details—such as which infections should be monitored, what measures will be used and the exact definitions of those measures, how risk adjustment for different patient populations should be done, what sources will be used to collect data, and what resources hospitals will need to perform collection and reporting tasks—vary from state to state or have yet to be addressed. For example, as of 2003, Illinois hospitals were required to submit data on surgical site infections, ventilator-associated pneumonia, and central line–associated bloodstream infections; beginning in 2004, Pennsylvania hospitals reported on surgical site and device-associated infections. This lack of standardization calls into question the validity of any data reported, as well as the usefulness of reports to patients, employers, and insurers for making decisions about care providers, as well as to health care organizations trying to use data to improve performance.

Making a Start

Many health care organizations across the country already participate in the National Healthcare Safety Network (NHSN, formerly the National Nosocomial Infections Surveillance system), administered by the Centers for Disease Control and Prevention (CDC). This voluntary reporting system enables the collection, exchange, and integration of information on infectious and noninfectious adverse events in health care settings. In February 2005 the CDC's Healthcare Infection Control Practices Advisory Committee released recommendations for designing and implementing public reporting systems for HAIs. Although the committee did not find enough scientific evidence to endorse or reject mandatory public reporting, they did come up with a set of recommendations based on established principles for public health and HAI surveillance. "I think the main message in the guideline is to encourage [policymakers] to use existing standards and either outcome or process measures that are already being recommended or required by other groups, such as the Centers for Medicare & Medicaid Services [CMS] or The Joint Commission," to design and implement a reporting system, says Denise Cardo, M.D., director of the CDC's Division of Healthcare Quality Promotion. "They really need to work with the groups that are involved in this issue," says Cardo.

The recommendations—which were developed in collaboration with the Association for Professionals in Infection Control and Epidemiology (APIC), the Society for Healthcare Epidemiology of America (SHEA), and the Council for State and Territorial Epidemiologists—comprise four main points,[1] as follows:

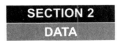

- Use of established public health surveillance methods. When establishing an HAI reporting system, policymakers should employ the following strategies: use appropriate process and outcome measures, as well as appropriate patient populations, for monitoring; standardized methods for case finding and validation of data; adequate support and resources; risk adjustment based on populations (underlying infections); and reports that have scientific meaning while still being understandable and useful to all stakeholders.
- Creation of a multidisciplinary advisory panel. Stakeholders should build a team that includes experts in infection control and prevention, which should oversee the planning and implementation of the reporting system.
- Choice and implementation of appropriate measures. Process and/or outcome measures should be chosen based on the type of facility, and they should be phased in gradually. The guidelines propose process measures addressing central line insertion practices, surgical antimicrobial prophylaxis, and influenza vaccination of patients/residents and health care workers, as well as outcome measures for central line–associated laboratory-confirmed primary bloodstream infections and surgical site infections (*see* Figure 11-1). Chapter 5 of this book, "Monitoring Patient Safety in Health Care: Building the Case for Surrogate Measures," pages 71–81, discusses the use of another type of reliable evaluation—clinically relevant surrogate measures.
- Provision of confidential feedback to health care providers. Policymakers should make sure the system includes a way for health care organizations to receive feedback confidentially. Regular reviews of performance data may help organizations target their prevention activities in problematic areas.

The guideline specifically advises against using hospital discharge diagnostic codes as the only source for HAI data. The complete guidance document for public reporting of HAIs can be accessed on the CDC's Web site at http://www.cdc.gov/ncidod/hip/PublicReportingGuide.pdf.

Moving Forward

The response to the recommendations from state policymakers has been positive. "We received several invitations to go to the states that had implemented or were considering implementing legislation to discuss the pros and cons of the specific outcome or process measures and to see if the NHSN would be a helpful tool for them," explains Cardo. The next critical step is to try to align the measures presented within the guideline with those already in use. "We're working with CMS to make sure that we are really recommending the same thing. That's the work we are doing right now—comparing the details."

It's the details that can make or break the reliability of any data collected, including the rates for specific infections. Hospitals often have conflicting views on which infections require data collection, which patients should be included, and so forth. These disparities mean that data from different hospitals aren't comparable. "It takes a lot of work to align measures," notes Nancy Lawler, associate project director in The Joint Commission's Division of Research. "A small wording difference in a data definition can make a big difference in what someone's rates look like. And it's not just the definitions of numerators and denominators; it's also who's included in your population and who's excluded."

Researchers continue to study standardized measures and processes, as well as the benefits and disadvantages of mandatory public reporting. For example, the National Quality Forum has initiated a project designed to standardize performance measures that can be used across all health care settings for the public reporting of HAIs. The project addresses four important areas: intravascular catheters and bloodstream infections, indwelling catheters and urinary tract infections, ventilators and respiratory infections, and surgical site infections.[2] The last area, surgical site infections, also appears as one of the four target areas of the Surgical Care Improvement Project (SCIP), a national partnership of organizations launched by CMS and CDC to improve the safety of surgical care by reducing postoperative complications.[4] SCIP currently includes six process measures for infections. In January 2006 APIC, SHEA, and the Infectious Diseases Society of America released model legislation to give state governments a template for HAI reporting systems. The model legislation's purpose is to ensure that state systems follow recommended practices to reduce the risks of HAIs, protect the confidentiality of medical records, and allow for differing degrees of illness in patient populations.[5]

No matter what standards and reporting systems may be developed, the push to reduce and prevent HAIs will keep gaining strength among stakeholders across the health care continuum. ∎

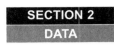

FIGURE 11-1. CDC–Recommended Measures for Mandatory Public Reporting of Health Care–Associated Infections[1]

Event	Measures	Rationale for Inclusion	Potential Limitations
Process Measures			
Central line insertion (CLI) practices	**Two measures (expressed as a percentage)** *Numerators:* Number of CLIs in which: • Maximal sterile barrier precautions were used • Chlorhexidine gluconate (preferred), tincture of iodine, an iodophor, or 70% alcohol was used as skin antiseptic *Denominator:* Number of CLIs	Unambiguous target goal (100%). Risk adjustment is unnecessary. Proven prevention effectiveness: Use of maximal barrier precautions during insertion and chlorhexidine skin antisepsis have been shown to be associated with an 84% and 49% reduction in central line–associated bloodstream infection rates, respectively.	Methods for data collection not yet standardized. Manual data collection likely to be tedious and labor intensive, and data are not included in medical records.
Surgical antimicrobial prophylaxis (AMP)	**Three measures (expressed as a percentage)** *Numerators:* Number of surgical patients: • Who received AMP within 1 hour prior to surgical incision (or 2 hours if receiving vancomycin or fluoroquinolone) • Whose prophylactic antibiotics were discontinued within 24 hours after surgery end time *Denominator:* All selected surgical patients	Unambiguous target goal (100%). Risk adjustment is unnecessary. Proven prevention effectiveness: • Administering the appropriate antimicrobial agent within 1 hour before the incision has been shown to reduce surgical site infections (SSIs). • Prolonged duration of surgical prophylaxis (> 24 hrs) has been associated with increased risk of antimicrobial-resistant SSI.	Manual data collection may be tedious and labor intensive, but data can be abstracted from medical records.
Influenza vaccination of patients and health care personnel	**Two measures (each expressed as a percentage of coverage)** *Numerators:* Number of influenza vaccinations given to eligible patients or health care personnel *Denominators:* Number of patients or health care personnel eligible for influenza vaccine	Proven prevention effectiveness: Vaccination of high-risk patients and health care personnel has been shown to be effective in preventing influenza.	Manual data collection may be tedious and labor intensive.
Outcome Measures			
Central line–associated laboratory-confirmed primary bloodstream infection (CLA-LCBI)	*Numerator:* Number of CLA-LCBIs *Denominator:* Number of central-line days in each population at risk, expressed per 1,000 *Populations at risk:* Patients with central lines cared for in different types of intensive care units (ICUs) *Risk stratification:* By type of ICU *Frequency of monitoring:* 12 months per year for ICU with < 5 beds; 6 months per year for ICU with > 5 beds *Frequency of rate calculation:* Monthly (or quarterly for small ICUs) for internal hospital quality improvement purposes *Frequency of rate reporting:* Annually using all the data to calculate the rate	Overall, an infrequent event but one that is associated with substantial cost, morbidity, and mortality. Reliable laboratory test available for identification (i.e., positive blood culture). Prevention guidelines exist, and insertion processes can be monitored concurrently. *Sensitivity:* 85%; predictive value positive (PVP): 75%. Low-frequency event but one that is associated with substantial cost, morbidity, and mortality.	LCBI can be challenging to diagnose because the definition includes criteria that are difficult to interpret (e.g., single-positive blood cultures from skin commensal organisms may not represent true infections). To offset this limitation, a system could include only those CLA-LCBIs identified by criterion 1, which will result in smaller numerators and therefore will require longer periods of time for sufficient data accumulation for rates to become stable/meaningful.
Surgical site infection	*Numerator:* Number of SSIs for each type of operation *Denominator:* Total number of each specific type of operation, expressed per 100 *Risk stratification:* Focus on high-volume operations and stratify by type of operation and National Nosocomial Infections Surveillance SSI risk index *Alternative risk adjustment:* For low-volume operations, by standardized infection ratio	Prevention guidelines exist, and certain important processes can be monitored concurrently. *Sensitivity:* 67%; PVP: 73%.	Standard definition of central line requires knowing where the tip of the line terminates, which is not always documented and can therefore lead to misclassification of lines. SSI definitions include a "physician diagnosis" criterion, which reduces objectivity. Rates dependent on surveillance intensity, especially completeness of postdischarge surveillance (50% become evident after discharge and may not be detected).

Reference
1. McKibben L., et al.: Guidance on public reporting of healthcare-associated infections: Recommendations of the Healthcare Infection Control Practices Advisory Committee. *Am J Infect Control* 33(4):217–226, 2005.

References

1. McKibben L., et al.: Guidance on public reporting of healthcare-associated infections: Recommendations of the Healthcare Infection Control Practices Advisory Committee. *Am J Infect Control* 33(4):217–226, 2005.

2. National Quality Forum (NQF): *National Consensus Standards for the Reporting of Healthcare-Associated Infection Data* [NQF project brief]. Nov. 2005. http://www.qualityforum.org (accessed Jan. 22, 2006).

3. Reduction in central line–associated bloodstream infections among patients in intensive care units—Pennsylvania, April 2001–2005. *MMWR* 54:1013–1016, Oct. 14, 2005.

4. MedQIC: *Surgical Care Improvement Project.* http://www.medqic.org/scip/ scip_homepage.html (accessed Jan. 23, 2006).

5. Association for Professionals in Infection Control and Epidemiology (APIC): *APIC, IDSA, SHEA Develop Model Legislation on Public Reporting of Healthcare-Associated Infections* [press release]. APIC, Jan. 23, 2006.

This chapter is modified from its original form in the newsletter *The Joint Commission Benchmark,* Volume 8, Number 2, March/April 2006, pp. 7–9 for inclusion in this book.

Ensuring the Use of Sterilized and Disinfected Equipment: Improving Infection Control While Reducing Turnaround Time and Costs

ASSESSMENT AND PRACTICE

Any medical device that comes in contact with a patient, regardless of the setting, has the potential for transmitting disease if it is not properly sterilized or disinfected after each use. Even something as simple as a blood pressure cuff can transmit microorganisms if it is not cleaned regularly. In addition, it is important to recognize when to take equipment out of service—that is, when disinfecting or sterilizing would be ineffective because the equipment is damaged or old. Keeping equipment clean in a safe, cost-efficient, and time-efficient manner can present a challenge in many organizations. But given the fact that more than two million hospital patients acquire health care–associated infections every year (*see* Chapter 14, "How Well Does Your Organization's Infection Control Program work?", page 137), the importance of using sterilized and disinfected equipment is clear. The following five suggestions can help your organization improve its methods of sterilizing and disinfecting equipment, while reducing turnaround time and costs.

Know the Classifications of Equipment and the Requirements for Cleaning Each Classification

In 1968 Earle Spaulding developed a classification system for patient care items and medical equipment that still guides disinfection and sterilization practices today. Spaulding's system classifies all medical equipment into the following three categories[1]:

- *Critical items* are those used in sterile body cavities. Such items include surgical instruments, cardiac and urinary catheters, implants, and ultrasound probes. They should be sterilized by steam, if possible, or treated with ethylene oxide, hydrogen peroxide gas, or liquid sterilants if they are heat sensitive.

- *Semicritical items* come in contact with mucous membranes or skin that is not intact. These items—including respiratory and anesthesia equipment, certain endoscopes, and laryngoscope blades—must receive at least high-level disinfection with chemical disinfectants.
- *Noncritical items,* such as bedpans, blood pressure cuffs, and bedrails, contact intact skin but not mucous membranes. They may be cleaned with low-level disinfectants.

Recommendations and guidelines for sterilization and disinfection of all categories of medical equipment are available from several agencies and associations, including the Centers for Disease Control and Prevention (CDC; http://www.cdc.gov), the Association of PeriOperative Registered Nurses (AORN; http://www.aorn.org), the Association for Professionals in Infection Control and Epidemiology (APIC; http://www.apic.org), the Association for the Advancement of Medical Instrumentation (AAMI; http://www.aami.org), the Food and Drug Administration (FDA; http://www.fda.gov), and the Environmental Protection Agency (EPA; http://www.epa.gov).

Clean All Equipment Before Sterilization or Disinfection

It is important to remember that if devices and equipment are not clean, they cannot be disinfected or sterilized. "Sterilants and disinfectants can't be effective if an item has proteinaceous material [blood, dirt, and so on] on it," explains Bonnie Barnard, surveillance epidemiologist for the Montana Department of Public Health and Human Services.

Follow Recommendations for Flash Sterilization Use

Many organizations use flash sterilization as a substitute for regular heat sterilization, even though guidelines published by the AAMI, AORN, and CDC all recommend limiting its use within specific clinical parameters, such as emergency situations in an operating room. Flash sterilization should be used only for patient care items that

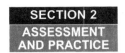
SECTION 2
ASSESSMENT
AND PRACTICE

CHAPTER 12 Ensuring the Use of Sterilized
and Disinfected Equipment: Improving Infection Control
While Reducing Turnaround Time and Costs

will be used immediately (such as to reprocess an instrument that was dropped accidentally); it should not be used for reasons of convenience. "Sometimes when people use a flash sterilizer, they neglect the normal procedures, so there's more potential for error," says Barnard. "You still have to use sterilizer indicators and keep records."

Use the Appropriate Disinfectant

Any staff member who cleans either medical equipment or environmental surfaces needs training to know what sterilization or disinfection products can be used for different items. The level of disinfectant—high, intermediate, or low—depends on the types of microorganisms that may be encountered and the types of body fluids to which the equipment has been exposed. For example, low-level disinfection destroys only vegetative bacteria and some fungi and viruses but not mycobacteria or spores; high-level, heat-automated disinfection destroys all microorganisms except high numbers of bacterial spores. Web sites for the EPA, FDA, CDC, and others provide recommendations for appropriate disinfectants in specific clinical situations.

Know the Amount of Equipment Available for Use and the Number of Procedures Performed when Determining Sterilization Needs

Scheduled procedures should not exceed equipment needs (except in emergencies only). There are advantages and disadvantages to any of the recognized sterilization technologies recommended for critical medical devices. For example, steam autoclaving is considered the gold standard but is time consuming, whereas some of the newer methodologies are faster but may be incompatible with certain materials (such as brass and copper) and lead to functional damage. Organizations need to remember these considerations when deciding on what technologies and products to use and purchase. For example, a hospital operating room that has a high patient turnover would likely invest in a steam sterilizer because the amount of equipment used and the number of procedures make it cost-effective. But this is not the case for every setting. "A clinic with a low turnover probably wouldn't have a steam sterilizer, but it may have equipment that requires sterilization," notes Barnard. "There are other alternatives for sterilization, such as peracetic acid. It all depends on the individual organization's needs."

For a description of a major medical center's success in reducing its rates of catheter-related blood stream infections and ventilator-associated pneumonia, see Chapter 1, "Eliminating Nosocomial Infections at Ascension Health," pages 9–24. ■

Reference

1. Rutala W.A., Weber D.J.: Disinfection and sterilization in health care facilities: What clinicians need to know. *Clin Infect Dis* 39:702–709, Sep. 1, 2004.

This chapter is modified from its original form in the newsletter *The Joint Commission Perspectives on Patient Safety™*, Volume 6, Number 11, November 2006, p. 11 for inclusion in this book.

Assessing and Addressing Infection Control Risks: How Does Your Organization Measure Up?

ASSESSMENT AND PRACTICE

When assessing the effectiveness of your organization's infection control (IC) program, consider asking yourself essential questions such as these: Do we have a program that assesses risks, sets priorities, determines objectives, and strives to meet those objectives? Does our organization measure the success of all IC initiatives and collect data to identify areas for further improvement? Most important, does our organization have a plan in place to respond to an outbreak of a health care–associated infection (HAI), and does it successfully carry out that plan when the situation warrants it? If you answered "no" to any of these questions, then your organization may be at risk for IC crisis.

Without an effective IC program, patients, staff, visitors, and volunteers can all be placed at risk for infection. Although contracting an infection may be just an inconvenience for some people, it can represent a life-threatening or fatal experience for others. Surgical site infections, bloodstream infections, and antibiotic-resistant infections can have serious consequences for patients, particularly those who are immunocompromised.

This chapter explores the components that make up an effective IC program, including the IC plan and surveillance activities. The chapter also shows the importance of communication and collaboration to the success of the plan. Next, it discusses areas of potential risk and provides tips and strategies to address those areas of risk. (Table 13-1 on page 125 contains a summary of the IC risks discussed in this article, along with possible solutions.) Finally, the chapter provides tips and suggestions on how to get leadership to champion your IC program so it can gain organizational status while benefiting from a generous allocation of resources.

Creating an Effective Infection Control Plan

An IC plan is a written document that discusses an organization's IC program. Joint Commission standards require organizations to have a written IC plan. Standard IC.1.10, element of performance (EP) 9 (*see* Box 13-1: Joint Commission Standards on Infection Control on page 123), outlines four basic components that every IC plan should have—a description of risks, a statement of goals, a description of strategies to address risks, and a description of how these strategies will be evaluated. "These four components should be the backbone of your organization's IC plan," says Louise Kuhny, an associate director in the Standards Interpretation Group of The Joint Commission. "They represent a continuous process improvement approach to managing IC risk." If any one of these components is missing, your plan will not meet Joint Commission standards, and, more important, your organization will be at risk for infection-related problems.

Contemplating Risks

When pondering potential IC risks, you need to carefully consider the characteristics of an organization, including its location, community environment, patient population, and the type of care, treatment, and services provided. "To help identify potential risks, organizations should communicate regularly with their public health department, as it can provide information and data on what IC issues are relevant within a particular community," says Kuhny. In addition to reviewing public health data, organizations should review and consider their own internal data when identifying IC risks.

> **TIP** **Make sure your IC plan has an appropriate scope.**
> Organizations should make sure that any IC plan covers not just patients and staff but all individuals who interact with the organization, including associates, physicians, students, contract workers, visitors, volunteers, and any others accessing the organization.

Prioritizing Risks and Setting Objectives

Because most organizations lack the resources to address every IC threat, it is important for them to prioritize such threats. "There are many ways to do this, including using criteria to rank the likelihood and seriousness of the threats. This could be a similar process to the one used to rank hazards in emergency management," says Kuhny.

SECTION 2
ASSESSMENT
AND PRACTICE

CHAPTER 13: Assessing and Addressing
Infection Control Risks: How Does Your
Organization Measure Up?

BOX 13-1. Joint Commission Standards on Infection Control

▶ **Standard IC.1.10** The risk of development of health care–associated infection is minimized through an organizationwide infection control program. This standard applies to the following programs: **ambulatory care, behavioral health care, critical access hospital, hospital, laboratory, long term care, office-based surgery,** and **home care.**

Element of Performance (EP) 6 ("Systems for the investigation of outbreaks of infectious diseases are in place") applies to the following programs: **ambulatory care, behavioral health care, critical access hospital, hospital, long term are,** and **home care.**

EP 9 ("The hospital has a written IC plan that includes the following: A description of prioritized risks; a statement of the goals of the IC program; a description of the hospital's strategies to minimize, reduce, or eliminate the prioritized risks; and a description of how the strategies will be evaluated") applies to the following programs: **ambulatory care, behavioral health care, critical access hospital, hospital, laboratory, long term care, office-based surgery,** and **home care.**

▶ **Standard IC.2.10** The infection control program identifies risks for the acquisition and transmission of infectious agents on an ongoing basis. This standard applies to the following programs: **ambulatory care, behavioral health care, critical access hospital, hospital, laboratory, long term care, office-based surgery,** and **home care.**

▶ **Standard IC.3.10** Based on risks, the hospital establishes priorities and sets goals for preventing the development of health care–associated infections within the hospital. This standard applies to the following programs: **ambulatory care, behavioral health care, critical access hospital, hospital, laboratory, long term care, office-based surgery,** and **home care.**

▶ **Standard IC.4.10** Once the organization has prioritized its goals, strategies must be implemented to achieve those goals.

EP 1 ("Interventions are designed to incorporate relevant guidelines for infection prevention and control activities.") applies to the following programs: **ambulatory care, behavioral health care, critical access hospital, hospital, laboratory, long term care, office-based surgery,** and **home care.**

▶ **Standard IC.5.10** The infection control program evaluates the effectiveness of the infection control interventions and, as necessary, redesigns the infection control interventions. This standard applies to the following programs: **ambulatory care, behavioral health care, critical access hospital, hospital, laboratory, long term care, office-based surgery,** and **home care.**

▶ **Standard IC.6.10** As part of emergency management activities, the organization prepares to respond to an influx, or the risk of an influx, of infectious patients. This standard applies to the following programs: **ambulatory care, behavioral health care, critical access hospital, hospital, laboratory, long term care,** and **home care.**

Source: The Joint Commission.

But setting priorities once without regularly revisiting the plan can open the organization up to increased risk. Your organization should review its IC plans, including its priorities, at least annually, and certainly when a problem, such as an outbreak, arises. It can be very helpful to involve a multidisciplinary team, such as an IC committee, in this process. "Organizations should keep a copy of the annual IC goals posted in a prominent place in the IC department so the IC team can regularly review them," says Terra Suriano, R.N., M.S.N., C.I.C., infection control coordinator for Advocate-Lutheran General Hospital in Park Ridge, Illinois.

Setting Goals That Address IC Risk Priorities

After setting risk priorities, create goals that address those priorities. Without goals—and plans to meet them—an organization cannot mitigate risks or improve the safety and quality of care. When determining goals and objectives for an IC program, you may want to look at your mission statement for the current year and build off that. "Organizations should also keep in mind what is mandated by regulation or standards of performance, as well as elements that are unique to the facility," says Suriano. Having a multidisciplinary group participate in goal development can be beneficial to the process.

Collecting Surveillance Data

An important aspect of any effective IC program is surveillance. This process involves collecting data about infections to identify risks, areas of improvement, and outbreaks. Surveillance data can show whether a process that was put in place to address risk is successful or whether further work is necessary. Because infection risks change over time, data collection must be ongoing.

Surveillance activities should include a review of all mandatory reporting data, such as information required by local, state, and federal agencies, and should reflect the priorities an organization has set for itself. "If your surveillance strategy does not reflect your organization's identified risks, then you are just collecting data to collect data," says Kuhny. "When your organization revises its IC priorities, the data collection strategy should also be revised accordingly."

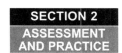

SECTION 2
ASSESSMENT
AND PRACTICE

CHAPTER 13: Assessing and Addressing
Infection Control Risks: How Does Your
Organization Measure Up?

TABLE 13-1. Infection Control (IC) Risks and Possible Solutions

IC Risk	Possible Solution
Health care–associated	Have a response plan in place that involves immediate infection outbreak response, education, and data monitoring.
No risk assessment or risk priorities in the IC plan	Assemble a multidisciplinary team to identify risks, considering the organization's geographic location, community environment, patient populations, and services provided, as well as relevant surveillance data.
IC plan does not reflect priorities.	Revise your plan to reflect identified risks. Your priorities should be posted where IC staff can easily see them. You should also review them regularly.
No measurable objectives or evaluation of objectives for the IC plan	Work with the multidisciplinary group to establish goals that reflect the organization's priorities. Data collection should allow you to measure how the organization meets its goals.
Lack of communication and collaboration between departments about IC issues	Establish IC as an organizationwide initiative. Leadership from every part of your organization should be involved in IC activities. If possible, IC professionals should sit on committees throughout the organization.
Minimal data collection	Collect data that help identify risks, respond to issues, determine the effectiveness of IC initiatives, and comply with local, state, and federal regulations.
Inadequate resources allocated to the IC program	Ask leadership to devote sufficient resources to the IC program. Use creative staffing solutions, such as hiring contract employees, to ensure adequate staffing.

Source: The Joint Commission.

The Most Effective Ways to Collect IC Data

After your organization decides what data it is going to collect, it must then determine how to collect it. There are a variety of effective ways to collect data. The following methods have been found to be effective:

- **Reporting systems.** These systems allow staff to phone, e-mail, or write reports about patients with infections. When a cluster of infections is reported, IC professionals, along with leadership, should take immediate action to address the outbreak and control its spread. Reporting systems might use a passive approach to surveillance that relies on health care or laboratory personnel to report issues. But if your organization wants to overcome the underreporting of issues, it must make it easy for staff to report them. It must not punish staff who report problems, by blaming them for the issues, and it must respond to the issues as reported.
- **Record review.** There are a variety of records from which your organization can collect data about infections, including admission logs, employee health records, incident reports, laboratory reports, patient records, pharmacy records, reports on the numbers and types of diagnostic workups and care recipient disposition, and treatment plans.
- **Rounds.** IC staff can engage in periodic rounds to consult with staff and make clinical observations. IC staff may also review charts, lab reports, and other relevant materials during this time.
- **Surveys.** These sources can include surveys of staff or patients. For example, in some organizations such as ambulatory facilities, telephone surveys can be valuable ways of collecting information from the patient after he or she has returned home. When an infection is suspected, staff can ask the patient to return to the organization for examination.
- **Literature reviews.** Although internal data are important to the discovery of infections, IC professionals should also keep an eye on the IC literature to find out about HAIs that are occurring or emerging in other organizations. Reliable sources for this type of information include:
  - The Association for Professionals in Infection Control and Epidemiology
  - The Centers for Disease Control and Prevention (CDC)
  - The Society for Healthcare Epidemiology of America
  - World Heath Organization

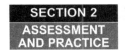

SECTION 2
ASSESSMENT
AND PRACTICE

CHAPTER 13: Assessing and Addressing
Infection Control Risks: How Does Your
Organization Measure Up?

- *Infection Control and Hospital Epidemiology*
- *Morbidity and Mortality Weekly Report*
- *American Journal of Infection Control*
- *OR Manager*
- Other IC professionals in your area

From such research, your IC professionals can determine whether your organization should be collecting internal data on these new infections and what control measures may need to be put in place.

TIP **Consider using technology to help review records for surveillance.**
Your organization can review records for surveillance measures through automated means or manually, depending on the size and scope of your organization's activities. Computers and software significantly ease the data collection process. Although data can be collected manually, electronic programs can sort and analyze data and generate rates, graphs, charts, and reports. Data can even be collected electronically through equipment such as personal digital assistants or scanning wands.

Identifying Trends

After the data have been collected, your organization must analyze the data, looking for trends, patterns, or significant issues that require attention. One proven way to do this is to benchmark the data. Internal benchmarking involves looking at data over time and/or comparing the data to other departments in the organization. Internal benchmarking can help your organization determine whether IC efforts are working to reduce infections and which areas still need attention.

External benchmarking enables your organization to compare itself against others to better evaluate problematic areas, as well as areas of success. Organizations can benchmark themselves against similar settings and against national databases such as the CDC's National Nosocomial Infections Surveillance system (which examines infection rates in adult and pediatric intensive care units, high-risk nurseries, and surgical patients) or the Surgical Infection Prevention Project (which analyzes antibiotic selection, administration, and discontinuation in surgical patients).

To effectively benchmark internal or external data, your organization should use measures that have standardized and uniform definitions and methods for data collection and risk adjustment. These measures allow your organization to compare like settings and get an accurate picture of how well your IC program is doing.

> **TIP** **If benchmarking reveals that goals are not being met, your organization must take steps to meet them.**
> If goals are not being met, you can resolve this problem through an improvement initiative. For example, all organizations are required by The Joint Commission to monitor their adherence to CDC hand hygiene guidelines. But simply collecting data is not enough. Your organization should set a specific goal for compliance and monitor the hand hygiene data to ensure that your organization meets its goal. If it does not, then initiatives, such as staff education, conveniently placed hand rub containers, and so forth, should be implemented to meet the goal. Data must again be collected to monitor the success of any new initiatives.

Responding to an HAI

The best way to respond to an HAI outbreak is to have a preset plan. "Standard IC.1.10, EP 6,* requires organizations to have a system set up ahead of time that outlines how an organization will respond to an outbreak. If your organization has not considered a response plan, then your organization cannot effectively and efficiently respond to an outbreak situation," says Kuhny.

Some things to consider when developing a response plan include when to activate the plan and what steps to take to control the outbreak. "Regular monitoring of laboratory data and patient/associate symptoms of illness can keep your finger on the pulse of your facility," says Suriano. "If an IC professional suspects an increase in cases, he or she must come up with a definition of the infection and then determine who meets that definition." The IC professional should also decide how many cases will define an outbreak; it could be as few as two or three depending on the illness. As soon as the IC professional becomes aware of an

---

* IC.1.10, EP 6 applies to **ambulatory care, behavioral health care, critical access hospital, hospital long term care,** and **home care**

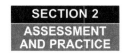
SECTION 2
ASSESSMENT
AND PRACTICE

CHAPTER 13: Assessing and Addressing
Infection Control Risks: How Does Your
Organization Measure Up?

outbreak, he or she should notify the clinical areas involved. "Face-to-face contact—talking with the staff about practice and procedure and then spending time observing practice—is really important," says Suriano. "The staff oftentimes can speak to the practice, but then during observation you find something a little different is being done."

Communicating and Collaborating About IC Issues

Establishing an effective IC program is not a one-time event. It requires continuous involvement of all organization staff, sustained leadership support, collaboration between departments, continuing staff education, and an evidence-based focus that incorporates new developments in the field. Without such efforts, an organization can fall short of its infection control and prevention goals and put itself at risk for IC–related incidents.

The successful creation of an organizationwide IC program requires collaboration to effectively collect and interpret data, design and implement interventions, and respond to outbreaks and other identified risks. Every area in your organization, including administration, medical staff, nursing units, building maintenance, food services, housekeeping, laboratory, pharmacy, and sterilization services, must work together to keep the IC program robust and responsive.

"Infection control practitioners should include themselves in organization committees, where possible, especially patient safety and physician driven quality committees," says Suriano. "Being involved in these types of committees allows the IC professional to bring IC data forward for the purpose of process improvement and enables the IC professional to hear about quality-related issues that may involve IC."

In addition to participating on committees, IC professionals need to maintain an open line of communication with organization leadership. "They should be involved in not only developing or revising IC policies, but also be an endorser of policies and procedures which contain components of IC and are developed by other departments," says Suriano.

Allocating Resources to IC

Although organizationwide involvement is crucial to the success of an IC program, dedicated IC professionals are needed to manage the day-to-day operations, identify areas of improvement, and respond to any issues that arise. In addition, other resources, such as computer equipment and supplies, must be allocated to the program. To determine the resources for an IC program, organizations should consider several factors, including the following:

- The type of care, treatment, and services the organization provides
- The characteristics of the patient population regarding IC
- Economic pressures and financial considerations

One way to balance IC needs with a tight budget is to hire an IC professional on a contractual basis. This person could be in charge of program design, administration, and evaluation but rely on other staff members to do the data collection. For further ideas on boosting the resources available to your IC program, *see* Chapter 15, "Making the Business Case for Infection Control," on pages 143–149.

Strategies and Tips for Achieving a Dynamic and Comprehensive IC Program

The success of your IC program rests on your ability to garner and maintain leadership support, educate staff members, ensure that IC risks in the environment are addressed, and keep abreast of new developments in the field. The following strategies and tips are aimed at making IC a priority for your entire organization every day, not just during targeted evaluations. A listing of some more IC risks and possible solutions can be found in Table 13-2 on page 134.

Engaging Medical, Nursing, and Executive Leadership

IC efforts do not only reside in the IC department. An organization can have a well-conceived IC plan and a hard-working IC staff, but if direct care staff members do not regularly wash their hands, if housekeeping staff members do not disinfect areas properly, or if nurses, physicians, and other staff members do not identify and isolate infectious patients, then the IC program cannot effectively prevent the

SECTION 2
ASSESSMENT AND PRACTICE

CHAPTER 13: Assessing and Addressing
Infection Control Risks: How Does Your
Organization Measure Up?

spread of infection. "Because IC is an organizationwide process, leaders who manage the people performing care, treatment, and services must be engaged in IC efforts and ensure that the organization's IC plan is effectively carried out," says the Standards Interpretation Group's Kuhny. "Leaders must integrate IC into their departments and encourage the staff to embrace IC initiatives."

 Leaders should give the IC program visible support and should actively participate in improving and strengthening it.

Here are some ways leaders can be asked to actively and visibly support an IC program:

- Allocate the resources necessary for a successful program. These resources include the appropriate number and skill mix of IC professionals, the time for all staff members to participate in IC education programs, and the proper equipment for IC practices—such as conveniently placed alcohol-based hand rub dispensers.
- Attend meetings on relevant IC issues and act as a consultative resource to the IC department.
- Publicly acknowledge successes in infection prevention and control, such as reduced health care–associated infections or decreased lengths of stay.
- Serve as a role model for good IC practices, such as effective hand hygiene or using appropriate barrier protections.
- Set expectations for the staff, such as following IC policies, requiring attendance at IC training programs, and following established hand hygiene guidelines.
- Support paying the staff for attending off-shift in-services or education sessions.
- Make IC procedures part of performance evaluations and competency reviews.

Educating Staff About IC Issues

One important way to give infection prevention and control an organizationwide focus is through ongoing staff education. Staff members must often change their behaviors to consistently implement IC practices, and you may not be able to change such behaviors during just one in-service. Your organization should consider offering IC–related education on the following topics:

- What individuals can do to prevent or control infection transmission
- How to identify current or potential IC problems
- How to report issues, including what to report, and to whom to report
- How to follow specific IC protocols and processes, including hand hygiene, patient isolation, and proper cleaning techniques

"There are some specific types of education that relate to IC that are required by the Occupational Safety and Health Administration (OSHA), including education on blood-borne pathogens and tuberculosis," says Kuhny. "Organizations should check OSHA and local and state regulations to ensure that they are providing any required education."

All staff members should receive IC education, including direct-care and clinical staff, as well as any other staff members who might come in contact with patients, such as biomedical technicians, food service staff, housekeeping staff, and delivery personnel.

 Your organization should vary not only the content of IC education, but also the venue at which the information is delivered.

Use the following suggestions to vary the education of your staff about IC issues:
- Regular in-services on topics such as hand washing
- Notices and flyers posted in staff break rooms or bathrooms
- Handouts and pamphlets about particular topics, such as chicken pox, West Nile virus, or hand-washing techniques
- Including the IC program in new staff orientation
- Newsletter articles that deal with IC topics, such as the flu season or disaster preparedness
- Regular visits from an IC practitioner with on-the-spot training
- Emergency management exercises

The Role of IC in the Environment of Care

Collaboration is a key component of a successful IC program. Although the IC department should communicate and collaborate with most departments in your organization, it is particularly important that the IC and environment of care (EC) departments have a strong working relationship.

To help ensure that IC issues are addressed in the environment, IC staff should participate on EC committees, such as those that set policies for cleaning, equipment maintenance, and building design and construction. There should be an open dialogue between the IC and EC departments to ensure that no aspect of the environment that relates to IC is overlooked. If IC staff does not have a presence on EC committees, or if the IC and EC departments do not communicate effectively with each other, then the opportunity for risk increases.

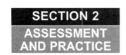

SECTION 2
ASSESSMENT
AND PRACTICE

CHAPTER 13: Assessing and Addressing
Infection Control Risks: How Does Your
Organization Measure Up?

PREPARING FOR AN IC EMERGENCY

Standard IC.6.10 requires organizations to prepare for an influx or the risk of an influx of infectious patients. An IC emergency is a lot like any other disaster—it can be unpredictable and has the potential of swamping an organization's care capabilities. Within the EC standards, The Joint Commission requires organizations to plan for emergencies by identifying and implementing actions that will help mitigate, prepare for, respond to, and recover from such events. Issues such as where to isolate infectious patients, how to quickly set up decontamination stations, and how to communicate effectively with public health agencies will all need to be considered in advance from both an IC and EC perspective.

 Establishing a relationship between the EC and IC departments before an emergency can help ensure an effective response to any IC–related situation.
IC staff members should participate in organization and community emergency management meetings, attend any multidisciplinary groups that identify hazards for the organization, work with their EC counterparts to create IC–specific emergency response plans, and coordinate exercises to test these plans. "Although The Joint Commission does not require organizations to integrate their IC and EC emergency management plans, many organizations choose to do so because the response to these types of emergencies can be quite integrated," says Kuhny.

 Emergency management plans are only as good as your staff's ability to carry them out.
Conducting exercises not only enables staff members to understand their role in responding to an IC emergency but also ensures that your organization plans for staff safety during an IC emergency. "If staff members don't feel they and their families are safe, they may not report to work during an IC emergency. So, exercises should not only address how staff members will take care of patients but also how their own safety will be addressed," says Kuhny.

Creating an Evidence-Based Program

To be effective, your IC program should reflect current practices within the field of IC. "Organizations should keep abreast of developments in the field and ensure that any IC plans reflect those developments," says Kuhny. For example, standard

TABLE 13-2. More Infection Control (IC) Risks and Possible Solutions

IC Risk	Possible Solution
Medical, nursing, and executive leadership not engaged in IC efforts	Encourage all levels of leadership to visibly and actively support IC efforts by participating in meetings, publicly sharing IC data, serving as role models for IC practices, or making IC practices part of the competency and review process for the staff.
Lack of staff education about IC	Provide education to all staff members regularly, and in a variety of formats.
IC staff not involved in environment of care (EC) issues	Ask IC professionals to develop a good working relationship with the EC department. They should be active in emergency planning efforts and have input on any EC policies that deal with IC risks.
IC staff do not play active roles in EC communities.	Participate on EC committees and develop open communication with EC leaders. Encourage IC professionals to make sure that IC issues in the environment are not overlooked.
Staff do not integrate the latest information about IC into the organization's processes to ensure an evidence-based program.	IC leadership should become aware of current IC issues throughout the country by working with the local public health department, collaborating with other IC professionals, and monitoring IC–related literature. IC leadership should then communicate this knowledge to all staff on a regular basis.

Source: The Joint Commission.

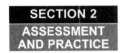

CHAPTER 13: Assessing and Addressing
Infection Control Risks: How Does Your
Organization Measure Up?

IC.4.10, EP 1, requires organizations to incorporate relevant guidelines within all IC activities. Relevant guidelines include those offered by the CDC, the Healthcare Infection Control Practices Advisory Committee, and the National Quality Forum. "Organizations should make sure their IC plans incorporate these guidelines when relevant," says Kuhny.

To stay on top of developments in the IC field, your organization can take the following steps:

- Build a relationship with the local public health department.
- Communicate and collaborate with other infection control practitioners in the field.
- Review literature and information that discusses IC issues.

TIP **Use reliable sources for IC information.**
Reliable sources include the CDC, the Association for Professionals in Infection Control and Epidemiology, *Infection Control and Hospital Epidemiology,* the Society for Healthcare Epidemiology of America, *Morbidity and Mortality Weekly Report, American Journal of Infection Control,* and *OR Manager.*

Effective IC management is fundamentally a group effort. Organizations that maintain a focused and collaborative program not only reduce the likelihood of IC risks, but also keep patients and staff safe while improving the overall quality of care. ■

This chapter is modified from its original form in the newsletter *The Joint Commission: The Source™,* Volume 4, Number 9 (September 2006, pp. 1–10) and Volume 4, Number 10 (October 2006, pp. 1–10) for inclusion in this book.

How Well Does Your Organization's Infection Control Program Work?

ASSESSMENT AND PRACTICE

It is an unfortunate fact that patients who arrive at hospitals or surgical centers for one condition, often acquire unrelated infections or other disorders during their stay. This situation is not new, but it has taken on a new significance in the era of modern technology as more advanced and invasive surgical techniques and treatment regimens—complicated by an increase in patient acuity, as well as a nursing shortage—have heightened the risks of exposure to infection. Between 1975 and 1996, the incidence of health care–associated infections (HAIs) rose from 7.2 to 9.8 per 1,000 patient stays.[1] That means that between 5% and 10% of patients admitted to acute care hospitals—more than two million each year—acquire one or more infections while there, resulting in nearly 90,000 deaths.[1] According to the Centers for Disease Control and Prevention (CDC), a third of these deaths may have been preventable.[2]

However, as incredible as it may seem, some health care organizations are finding that they can reduce the incidence of HAIs to near zero using industrial process improvement techniques developed by companies such as Toyota. (*See* Chapter 3, "Using Real-Time Problem Solving to Eliminate Central Line Infections," pages 41–56, for practical information on implementing these techniques.)

One way that your health care organization can help prevent the spread of infection is by complying with Joint Commission Standard IC.5.10, which requires organizations to evaluate the effectiveness of their infection control program (IC) to determine which program activities are effective and which activities should be changed to improve outcomes. According to Louise Kuhny, an associate director in

The Joint Commission's Standards Interpretation Group, complying with this standard means that organizations must also comply with the requirements of related standards. "You can't look at IC.5.10 by itself," says Kuhny. "Standards IC.2.10 through IC.5.10 [*see* Box 13-1 on page 123] are all part of a continuum. If an organization is examining its infection control program and looks only at IC.5.10, it'll miss most of the picture. It needs to look at the entire program as a process of continuous improvement."

Kuhny cautions organizations to recognize and evaluate Standard IC.5.10 as the culmination of an infection control program that starts with Standard IC.2.10. "Standard IC.2.10 is really the foundation of the program because it concerns how the organization identifies the risks associated with infection control and infectious agents," says Kuhny.

In Standard IC.3.10, the organization is expected to establish goals. In Standard IC.4.10, the organization prioritizes those goals and develops and implements strategies; then, as required in Standard IC.5.10, organizations evaluate their infection control efforts.

"After organizations determine their risk, establish their goals and priorities, and implement their strategies, IC.5.10 requires them to stand back and evaluate to see how they're doing," says Kuhny. She suggests that organizations should ask themselves: Have our interventions been correct? Have they been effective? Do we need to reevaluate and determine whether different interventions would be more appropriate? Does the risk analysis need to be conducted again? Do we need to devote more resources to infection control? A number of important strategies can help your organization answer these questions, to better evaluate the effectiveness of its IC program.

Five Strategies to Help Assess Your Organization's Infection Control Program

STRATEGY 1: Evaluate whether changes need to be made to your organization's infection control program in light of emerging diseases by consulting sources such as the CDC.

As required by Standard IC.5.10, element of performance (EP) 1, organizations must conduct an evaluation of their infection control program at least annually and

SECTION 2
ASSESSMENT
AND PRACTICE

CHAPTER 14: How Well Does Your Organization's
Infection Control Program Work?

whenever risks change significantly. A change in risk can happen for a number of reasons, including the emergence of new diseases, such as severe acute respiratory syndrome (SARS) or West Nile fever. In addition to new diseases, organizations must also prepare for reemerging diseases, such as whooping cough. "Illinois experienced a whooping cough outbreak during each of the last two winters," says Kuhny, "so Illinois organizations needed to change their risk analyses and interventions." Another reemerging pathogen is measles, which has appeared recently in Indiana and Ohio, forcing organizations in those states to reexamine their current risks. To keep up to date on emerging and reemerging pathogens, as well as relevant infection control and prevention guidelines, consult the CDC's Web site at http://www.cdc.gov. You can also gather information on these topics from your state public health department, as well as from professional societies, such as the Society for Healthcare Epidemiology of America (http://www.shea-online.org) and the Association for Professionals in Infection Control and Epidemiology (http://www.apic.org). Try to incorporate the new guidelines, along with information from recent studies into your organization's policies and procedures.

STRATEGY 2: Reevaluate the effectiveness of your infection control program whenever your organization changes the scope of its services.

If your organization changes the scope of its services, introducing new services or new sites of care, you need to determine whether new infection risks have been created. For example, if your organization adds a wing to provide cardiac care, a Level III neonatal intensive care unit, or a Level I high-risk trauma center, you may need to make adjustments to its infection control protocols to protect patients in the new areas. "Those patients carry a different set of infection control risks than patients who are at a lower risk," says Kuhny.

STRATEGY 3: Use data collection and analysis to evaluate the effectiveness of your infection control program.

Standard IC.5.10, EP 5, requires organizations to evaluate the success or failure of their interventions. "This is where the circular nature of these standards is most apparent," says Kuhny. She points out that IC.2.10, EP 3, requires organizations to identify infection prevention and control risks by using surveillance activities, including the data collection and analysis of infections. The nature of the data collected under Standard IC.3.10 is determined by the risk assessment in Standard IC.2.10 and the goals established in Standard IC.3.10. The data should be analyzed by an individual who understands both the data themselves and the context in which they were collected. Standard IC.4.10 requires the organization to implement its intervention. Finally, Standard IC.5.10, EP 5, requires that organizations measure the effectiveness of the intervention, based on surveillance activities that are described in Standard IC.2.10. "Organizations looking at IC.5.10 should be measuring based on what they identified as risks in IC.2.10," says Kuhny, "It's really a performance improvement activity that keeps circling back on itself in a process of continuous improvement."

Your organization should conduct both external comparisons (with other organizations) against national benchmarks or published studies, and internal measurement (comparing the organization's performance over time). Many organizations use some kind of statistical analysis tool for these purposes. "Although The Joint Commission doesn't recommend any specific tool, the organization can choose tools such as run charts, control charts—anything where you can statistically analyze the data points over time to see how you're doing," says Kuhny. If your organization participates in the CDC's National Healthcare Safety Network, you can also use its collected data to see how your organization stacks up against other, similarly sized organizations nationally (*see* Chapter 11, "National Data Report: Hospital Infection Reporting Guidelines," pages 111–116).

STRATEGY 4: Welcome open communication about infection control so you can obtain valuable feedback about the effectiveness of your infection control program.

Your organization should make sure that staff feel comfortable voicing their concerns about infection control. Feedback can be gathered through tools such as surveys, focus groups, discussions, and hotlines. Whichever method you choose, make sure that it is easy for staff members to use.

"Although not all hospitals have infection control committees, they do have an infection control function. There should be a way to raise concerns and bring those concerns to the attention of the people who are responsible," says Kuhny.

By evaluating its infection control program, your organization can enhance the quality of care provided. It is crucial to make this evaluation an ongoing process to ensure that your organization adapts and changes in response to newly emerging infection risks.

SECTION 2
ASSESSMENT
AND PRACTICE

CHAPTER 14: How Well Does Your Organization's
Infection Control Program Work?

STRATEGY 5: Determine whether your IC program needs more resources to carry out its important functions.

Today's health care organizations face increasing demands in an era of diminishing resources. How can you obtain a larger IC budget and increase your staff in such an environment? Denise Murphy, R.N., M.P.H., CC.I.C., chief patient safety and quality officer at Barnes-Jewish Hospital in St. Louis, recommends thinking of your IC program as a business that can positively impact your organization's bottom line. See Chapter 15, "Making the Business Case for Infection Control," pages 143–149, for a explanation of how to obtain more resources for your IC program by showing leadership the program's essential function as a revenue enhancer. ■

References

1. Burke J.: Infection Control—A problem for patient safety. *New Engl J Med.* 348:651–656, Feb. 13, 2003.

2. Harbarth S., et al.: The preventable proportion of nosocomial infections: An overview of published reports. *J Hosp Infec.* 54:256–258, Aug. 2003.

This chapter is modified from its original form in the newsletter *The Joint Commission: The Source,* Volume 4, Number 3, March 2006, pp. 1, 2, 11 for inclusion in this book.

Making the Business Case for Infection Control

ASSESSMENT AND PRACTICE

Do you want more resources for your infection control (IC) program? Then show your health care executives that you understand their priorities by proving that a reduction in health care–associated infections (HAIs) will positively affect your organization's bottom line.

Using this business argument, Denise Murphy, R.N., M.P.H.,C.I.C., chief patient safety and quality officer at Barnes-Jewish Hospital (BJH) in St. Louis, was able to double the resources for the IC program over a five-year period. "The first year, we lowered bloodstream infections in one ICU. The next year, we did it in two more ICUs, and so on," she recalls. "We were also able to show the organization a return on its investment."

Defining the Mission and Setting the Goals

The first step in making the business case for infection control is to align the IC program and the organizational missions, says Murphy. To that end, you need to communicate a clear understanding of the reason your program exists. For example, the IC program at BJH has a mission "to improve the safety and quality of patient care by decreasing the impact of infections and exposures acquired throughout the health care continuum in a cost-effective manner." The IC program's aim to improve safety and quality and reduce costs got the executives' attention.

The next step is to set annual goals and objectives. A goal should state the desired purpose or aim, (for example, that the program will increase productivity by discontinuing total house surveillance and conducting focused surveillance for HAIs). Objectives are actions taken to meet specific goals. An example is that the IC committee will select criteria-based intensive care unit (ICU) surveillance indicators within a certain time frame.

Developing a vision is also helpful. "Creating a vision requires forward thinking and imagination," Murphy explains. "It outlines a dream for the future and commits everyone to a common cause." A vision includes short-term (one to three years) and long-term (the next five years and beyond) goals and objectives. "Linking the IC program's mission to the organization's mission shows the executives that you are leaders who understand the strategic imperatives and want to contribute to meeting the targets for key result areas," says Murphy, adding, "Your executives will look at you with a lot more respect because you understand the big picture."

The Impact of Health Care–Associated Infections

The best business argument for supporting IC programs (which includes adding resources, or defending against the cutting of resources) is educating health care executives about the clinical impact of HAIs. Here is some ammunition you can use to show the national impact of HAIs on the health care system:

- HAIs are the fourth leading cause of death in the United States.[1]
- Each year, 2.1 million HAIs occur.[2]
- For every 100 hospital admissions, 5.7 HAIs occur.[2]
- HAIs cause or contribute to about 90,000 deaths a year.[2]
- HAIs cause an excess length of stay of 7.5 million days.[2]
- HAIs cause excess expenses of more than $6 billion.[2]
- Mean cost per case attributed to bloodstream infections is $38,703.[2]
- Mean cost per case of an HAI related to methicillin-resistant *S. aureus* is $35,367.[2]

The sobering impact of occupational exposures on your organization's employees also makes a compelling argument. The following statistics are derived from the Centers for Disease Control and Prevention (CDC)[3]:

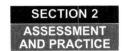
- An estimated 385,000 needlesticks and other sharps-related injuries are sustained by hospital-based health care personnel annually.
- On average, 1,000 sharps injuries occur daily.
- Eighty-four percent of all confirmed or potential HIV cases reported in health care workers are due to needlestick injuries.
- An estimated 500 health care workers are infected with the hepatitis B virus annually, despite an available vaccine.
- The average risk of hepatitis C virus transmission to an employee after needlestick exposure to an infected patient is 1.8%.

Although it's most effective to demonstrate the local impact of HAIs, Murphy says, it's not always easy to document the cost to an organization. She suggests setting up a case-control study to evaluate the costs of infection acquired during procedures, such as coronary artery bypass, that have fixed costs. This strategy is easier than looking at the cost of infections associated with medicine service admissions, where patients often have several comorbidities, a factor that introduces more cost variables. Compare the total costs of hospitalization for patients who didn't get an infection to those of patients who did. For the latter patients, don't forget to include costs incurred because of readmission, including a second surgical procedure, operating room (OR) time, ICU care, and additional medications. Murphy suggests asking someone in the accounting department to assist in the evaluation.

If obtaining organizational costs is not possible, Murphy suggests using cost estimates from the literature. The key is to adjust costs for health care inflation, which is currently at 4% annually. Adjusting 1999 costs up to 2005 costs requires multiplying each year's costs by the inflation rate. For example, adjusted for inflation, a bloodstream infection that cost $4,500 in 1999 costs $5,694 in 2005.

Hidden Costs

Explore the lost or hidden opportunity costs that result from HAIs as well. These costs refer to resources consumed for one purpose that are then unavailable for another, potentially higher-value activity, Murphy explains. If a significant amount of OR time is spent treating patients with complications of infections, fewer new surgeries may be performed during a given time period. Murphy warns that the potential to see profits from preventing HAIs depends on how your organization is reimbursed by insurers or third-party payers. A private insurance company may pay for all extra days spent in the hospital as a result of an HAI. Conversely, under a managed care contract, the hospital may receive only one fixed payment, regardless of the length of stay or the costs of treating a complication brought on by infection.

Balance the cost information with the understanding that many variable costs (costs that can change with patient census) are "sticky." Sticky costs don't change with patient census, so the actual reduction in operating costs from preventing HAIs is usually smaller than the numbers would suggest, Murphy cautions. For example, an ICU bed that is free because of fewer HAIs may still be used by a marginal candidate for the unit. Therefore, the anticipated cost savings in ICU care and supplies may not be realized from infection prevention. Similarly, staffing costs may not change, even if fewer patients with infections are receiving nursing care.

That's why it is important not to make cost savings from prevented HAIs the sole argument for IC programs, urges Murphy. IC programs benefit your organization well beyond the reduction of costs. Here are some additional IC benefits:

- Dedicated professionals who are focused on reducing adverse clinical outcomes
- Access to epidemiology and measurement skills applicable to other areas of a health care process or to quality improvement
- Eliminated waste and improved productivity through wise product selection oversight
- Input for the appropriate application of expensive technology and sensible policies and procedures.
- Protection of employees from injury
- Maintained regulatory compliance
- Effective collaboration in deploying evidence-based practices that prevent infections and medical errors
- A safer environment for patients and staff

The negative impact of HAIs also surfaces in declining patient referrals and the downgrading of your organization's reputation. These days, the public is much more aware of the risks of acquiring an infection in the hospital. "Once word gets out that

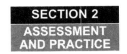

there's an outbreak, it can wreak havoc on the volume admitted to the particular service involved," Murphy says. Moreover, it is commonly held wisdom that keeping existing customers is far less expensive than attracting new ones, and that employees satisfied with their workplace are less likely to seek employment elsewhere.

Finally, it is important to remember that HAIs negatively affect your patients in several ways: indirect costs to their families and caretakers, lost years of productive life, emotional and social burdens, a lowered trust in the health care system, and the increased use of antibiotics, which can result in resistance problems.

A Cost-Effective Program

When building a case for increased resources to support an effective IC program, describe the program clearly, state who the IC practitioners are and what they do, and explain what the program expects to accomplish. You should also list the resources you need to implement the surveillance program effectively, establish performance improvement teams focused on reducing risk, and carry out those interventions that are proven to reduce HAIs. Let's look at these steps in more depth.

RESOURCES ALLOCATION

Allocate resources based on the following criteria:

- Population demographics
- Most common diagnoses
- High-risk populations
- Services offered
- Type and volume of procedures performed

According to the CDC's Delphi Project, the resources needed to support a typical IC program include one trained IC practitioner for every 100 occupied beds.[4] It is also essential to have a trained physician leader. The IC program at BJH consists of one IC manager, six full-time IC practitioners, one statistical analyst, one epidemiology technician, and one project coordinator to cover approximately 1,400 beds with an inpatient census of about 900 (occupied beds).

Other necessary resources include:

- Information systems (for example, computers, Internet access, integrated databases)
- Clerical, analytical, and statistical support
- Laboratory support (for example, money for gene typing)
- A dedicated budget (for example, money for education and professional development)

PERFORMANCE IMPROVEMENT TEAMS

As part of the overall program, establish performance improvement teams to implement HAI reduction interventions, but don't reinvent the wheel, Murphy urges. Instead, use the literature and tools that other organizations have perfected. Use credible data to create an urgency to drive such interventions, all of which should be evidence based.

FOCUSED SURVEILLANCE

Although conducting total house surveillance can be beneficial, it can also be cost-prohibitive, especially in larger institutions, Murphy says. "Conducting focused surveillance will enable you to get a handle on the organization's largest problems, which are high-risk, high-volume, or problem-prone infections," she adds. At BJH, the IC practitioners review all positive microbiologic cultures, using an automated surveillance system. Focused surveillance, with full chart review and investigation, is conducted for central venous catheter–related bloodstream infections, ventilator-associated pneumonia, and surgical site infections. Surgical site infections tracked at BJH include cardiac and orthopedic surgeries, neurosurgeries, and C-sections. BJH also tracks antibiotic-resistant organisms, such as methicillin-resistant *S. aureus,* vancomycin-resistant enterococci, and *Clostridium difficile.* Staff also monitor high-risk patient populations, such as oncology patients, for adverse events.

To keep data collection from becoming too burdensome, Murphy suggests using automated surveillance and requesting additional lab/clerical support, when necessary. Comparing your organization against others locally can offer a fresh—and sometimes alarming—perspective. Use the data available from the CDC's National Healthcare Safety Network to access such comparative data (*see* Chapter 11, "National Data Report: Hospital Infection Reporting Guidelines," pages 111–116). Murphy also recommends distributing an annual report with the IC program's goals for the coming year and trumpeting its previous accomplishments.

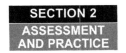

Murphy hopes that pay-for-performance programs will eventually include IC indicators as part of their measurement. National quality initiatives already look at bloodstream infections, the care of mechanically ventilated patients, and the use of surgical antibiotic prophylaxis, she notes. ■

References

1. Wenzel R.P., Edmond M.B.: The impact of hospital-acquired bloodstream infections. *Emerg Infect Dis* 7:174–177, Mar.–Apr. 2001. http://www.cdc.gov/ncidod/eid/vol7no2/wenzel.htm (accessed Jan. 25, 2007).

2. Graves N.: Economics and preventing hospital-acquired infection. *Emerg Infect Dis* 10:561–566, Apr. 2004. http://www.cdc.gov/ncidod/EID/vol10no4/02-0754.htm (accessed Jan. 25, 2007).

3. Centers for Disease Control and Prevention: Overview: Risks and prevention of sharps injuries in healthcare personnel. http://www.cdc.gov/sharpssafety/ (accessed Jan. 25, 2007).

4. O'Boyle C., Jackson M., Henly S.J.: Staffing requirements for infection control programs in US health care facilities: Delphi project. *AJIC* 30:321–333, Oct. 2002.

This chapter is modified from its original form in the newsletter *The Joint Commission Perspectives on Patient Safety,* June 2005, Volume 5, Number 6, pp. 1–4 for inclusion in this book.

Index

Pressure ulcer prevention, 31
Primum non nocere ("First, do no harm"), v
Private rooms. *See* Patient rooms
Process measures, 74–75, 79, 113–115
PSIC (Patient Safety Improvement Corps), 37
PUD (peptic ulcer disease), 19

Q

Quality and Patient Safety Awards (PHA), 31
Athens Regional Medical Center, 31–34
Habersham County Medical Center, 34–35
Systematic Assessment of Flow and Error (SAFE) tool, 32–34
Quality improvement, reporting systems for, 25
Quality Improvement Organization Programs (CMS), 110
Quality of care
    measures for, 71
        development of, 74, 79
        outcome measures, 113–115
        process measures, 74–75, 79, 113–115
        surrogate measures, 75–78, 79, 113
ORYX® performance measurement requirements, 107
Surgical Care Improvement Project (SCIP), 107–110, 114

R

Rapid action cycle, 64, 66
Respiratory SCIP process and outcome measures, 109

S

SAFE (Systematic Assessment of Flow and Error) tool, 32–34
SafeCare Committee, 31
Safe Medication Use (SMU), 30–31
SARS (Severe Acute Respiratory Syndrome) precautions, 104
SCIP (Surgical Care Improvement Project), 107–110, 114
Semmelweis, Ignaz, ix, xi
SENIC (Study on the Efficacy of Nosocomial Infection Control) Project, 72
Sentinel Event Database (Joint Commission), 32
Severe Acute Respiratory Syndrome (SARS) precautions, 104
Sharps injuries, 145
Society for Healthcare Epidemiology of America (SHEA), 112, 114, 139
Spaulding, Earle, 117
Staff
    champions for CR-BSI initiatives, 13, 22
    education of
        CL processes, 11–12, 44–45, 52–53
        IC issues, 131–132, 134
        VAP processes, 17–18, 21–22
    feedback on IC program, 140
    influenza vaccinations, 113, 114, 115